TANTRIC SEX:

THE ULTIMATE GUIDE TO POSITIONS FOR BEGINNERS AND ADVANCED COUPLES. TRANSFORM YOUR LIFE WITH SEXUAL TECHNIQUES AND SECRET TIPS FOR MEN AND WOMEN TO PLAY YOUR RELATIONSHIP GAMES

LAUREN RICHARDSON

CONTENT

INTRODUCTION

Before beginning with tantric sex, it is pivotal to comprehend the idea of Tantra. The act of Tantra can be followed back to antiquated India, where a few holy people and blessed men used to take part in different ceremonial and meditational systems. This system is accepted to have been in presence since the fifth century A.D., and it was seen as a technique that would enable an individual saddle to divine cognizance just as their still, small voice. This idea traversed the globe and brought about the cutting edge use of the term Tantra accepting another importance through and through. The term Tantra is prominently connected with the act of Tantric sex. This includes participating in a sexual demonstration with the purpose of collecting divine cognizance together. To lay it out plainly, tantric sex is a training that is used for arriving at sexual nirvana.

HISTORY OF TANTRA

There is some indefinite quality with respect to the birthplace of the idea of tantric sex, however it is a prevalent view that a network, alluded to as the "Lemurian" individuals were viewed as the primary individuals to rehearse this specific type of holy sex. They thought about the human body as an awesome vessel and used different animating procedures for connecting with the senses so as to bring in spiritual liberation. A few people will, in general, accept that Tantra is identified with the old Indian act of "yoga" too, since these two systems use distinctive substantial stances for shaping a bond with the Cosmos.

Tantric sex has increased a great deal of prevalence in the ongoing past and it has gotten well known in the western world with a ton of famous people like Sting, Madonna and even the late Steve Jobs who had confessed to having attempted this system. Presently, it has gradually discovered acknowledgment everywhere throughout the world. A few idealists do have faith in its viability in accomplishing more noteworthy delight.

Tantric sex fulfills individuals genuinely, intellectually and deeply too. Tantric sex gives total fulfillment and causes the whole body to feel incredibly pleasurable, helps in sincerely interfacing with one's partner and on a deep level; it helps in the amalgamation of two spirits and carries them closer to godliness.

Tantra uses two energies; the female and the male energies. The female energy is alluded to as Shakti, and the male energy is known as Shiva. Shakti and Shiva are Hindu divine beings, and their object of worship revere includes the venerating of Ling and Yon. Linga implies the penis and far off methods the vagina. When a couple participates in tantric sex, then the female energy present in the body, Shakti, ascends through the diverse chakras, and it penetrates through the female community that is alluded to as the Kundalini and afterward it converges with the male energy, alluded to as Shiva. This combination of energies helps in framing a bond that outperforms the human domain.

DIFFERENT PARTS OF TANTRIC SEX

There are three significant primary parts of Tantric sex, and these are tantric correspondence, tantric positions and tantric working out. Tantric correspondence is a procedure that helps in the converging of a couple genuinely and intellectually. This aids in bringing them near each other and is fit for transforming a standard couple into perfect partners. Tantric positions are sure places that will help in uniting a couple explicitly. There are distinctive tantric activities just as breathing strategies that will help in harvesting the most out of tantric sex. More data about these three parts of Tantric sex has been clarified in the coming sections.

Tantric sex helps in liberating the body, brain and soul. This is conceivable through the act of the systems as referenced previously. Quieting one's psyche is a vital part of any training that includes meditation. So also, for practicing tantric sex, it is basic to facilitate your brain. These procedures have been referenced in the book.

In contrast to normal sex, the lessons of tantric sex focus on making the members mindful of their activities while engaged with a sexual demonstration with their partner. If you are aware of your activities, then you can guarantee that you can initiate a sentiment of veneration and even regard for your partner. It is tied in with respecting your body and that of your partner's also. The essential goal of tantric sex is to assist you with loosening up your body and brain. When you can discover this discharge, you will have the option to communicate without any difficulty that will develop and reinforce the security that exists among you and your partner; the sort of love that would bind together your spirits.

TANTRIC SEX ENCOURAGES YOUR HEALING

Maybe one of the best potential employments of tantric sex is that it can help in healing your body and soul. It will likewise assist you with letting go of undesirable thoughts and cause your psyche to feel lighter. You may have been harmed before or might have persevered through some type of dismissal in your past connections. Tantric sex will help you in excusing yourself and will assist you with learning to adore yourself by and by and to appreciate your body as you were intended to. Various strategies have been referenced right now will help you in mending and liberating yourself from any blame or injury that you may have persevered. You will see that you will feel progressively engaged if you follow the guidance that has been given right now. Tantric sex will without a doubt, assist you with mending and it is done through the next advances. You should distinguish the occurrence that has harmed you previously. This hurt could have been genuine or nonexistent. In this way, the subsequent stage is to decide if it was genuine or fanciful. Sexual incitement will help you in recognizing the distinction. You will have the option to locate the negative feelings connected to this specific damage and can release them. Replace these negative sentiments with positive feelings and encounters that will enable you to heal.

UNDERSTANDING WHAT TANTRIC PHILOSOPHY IS

So, what's the philosophy behind tantric sex? It's quite interesting and very important to know. The philosophy behind this is simple to understand, and very effective to learn.

THE PURPOSE OF IT

Tantric sex has at a core a purpose that can help you improve your sex life. For most people, there are many goals and expectations that involve how we look at sex, and the way it should be done, along with habits and routines we must follow that make us feel like we're in a rut sexually.

Tantra is about taking all of that and throwing it out the window, so your ultimate goal is to not focus on the routines and habits of sex, but instead starting with a fresh and new look to it. This basically takes out the whole veteran aspects of it, assuming you know everything, and it lets you look at things almost like a beginner.

This refines sex in another way too. It makes it more about connection, intimacy, and the possibility of it that's playful and fun, rather than just racing to have an orgasm.

For most people, tantric sex has as one of the philosophies to learn and rediscover all of this for yourself. Let go of the concept where you have to just "get someone off" or achieve really anything. Once you do that, there's more room for discovery and a lot more fun.

You take out the whole thought process behind this, and instead, look at things in a personalized manner so you can benefit from it too.

LESS ABOUT THE THOUGHTS, MORE ABOUT THE MOMENTS

When we do things, we oftentimes are thinking only about the thoughts, rather than the moments we need to experience. That's why most of us struggle with orgasms because we're so hung up on trying to orgasm that sometimes we don't, or if we do, it's not that memorable or powerful.

But, with tantric sex, you're experiencing everything at the moment, including orgasms that are much more powerful, longer-lasting, a lot more non-ejaculatory, and also the full-body orgasms for both men and women.

That's because, it's less just about the genitalia orgasm, and more about the well, everything else orgasm.

The orgasms that you have are different. They are more about in the moment, where you're not focusing on the mechanics of life, but just well, what you're doing.

It brings a sort of oneness with life, and your partner, something that the Hindu religions try to go for.

While you're not trying to go for nirvana-like in Buddhism, but when you orgasm in a tantric manner, it basically lets you surrender your body, the states of vision, and promotes a oneness between you and the other person.

It's a very spiritual activity, and even those who are reacting it just in a secular manner do experience a glimpse of the divinity because of the melting of your regular self during those moments. When you experience this, it's almost like you're becoming a new, refined person, and in many cases, lets you push through the bad, and experience the good.

RELEASES SEXUAL BLOCKS

Tantric sex is great for releasing the sexual blocks, and the trauma that's there. Tantric sex targets your third chakra, which is located between the breastbone and navel, which is where your self-esteem is, and if it's out of balance, this can cause issues in bed.

When you work on the confidence you desire, you'll feel a stronger sense of resolve in yourself, and you'll quit shaming yourself and learn to love it.

Oftentimes, sexual blocks come about because of trauma in the past, and it's made us play the victim. That trauma, whether it be rape, or coercion or even just a toxic boyfriend that abused you, will cause this to fall out of whack, and sometimes, one of the sexual blocks we do have is choosing ourselves first.

Tantric sex helps you do this, and you need to learn that it's a valuable activity that lets you get over hose bonds.

Tantric sex is slow, sensual, and lets you really feel in the moment. For most people, they don't even realize they're held back by their past, which can mean that they're not doing what makes them happy. Instead, they're acting almost robotic, not working towards a better, more rewarding experience but instead playing the victim, thinking that they can't really benefit from sex.

But tantric sex can help you feel beautiful and worthy, and tantra encourages you to breathe into the third chakra, which in turn will help provide more and better energies too. You can say this to yourself during everything, and you'll affirm this over time.

Tantric sex also encourages you to get a deeper meaning of yourself, helping you overcome the issues you might have during sex, improving your own personal wellness, and understanding too.

NEOTANTRA ISN'T AS COMPLEX AS THE OTHERS

Classical tantra, of course, focuses more on the awakening and enlightenment, and this can happen, but it needs a more personalized and rigorous dedication, involves various meditative practices, and also might use more visualizations, mantras, and worshipping the deity. With classical tantra, sex isn't the focus.

But, the philosophy behind the neotantra, which developed in the last two centuries, is about fulfilling connection and intimacy, improving the connection between your emotions and the body, healing your trauma, and various blocks, and of course, reaching ecstasy in terms of orgasms.

It's much deeper than you'd think. This connection is just how you understand your emotions and body that you have. Most of us are held back because of past events. If you talk to people, they're held back by the pain that they've had before.

Men with erectile dysfunction, for example, might struggle because of self-esteem issues, and while opening the third charka is done by mantras and breathing, tantric sex lets them feel warm, welcomed, and can heal the trauma.

Many women experience issues with this too. Sexual concerns, especially with orgasm, are a very common thing, but with tantric sex, you start to connect these better and heal this, so you reach a better, greater sense of ecstasy and pleasure.

Some women are hung up on not experiencing orgasms in the past, but with tantric sex, it helps bring about the orgasmic ecstasy that they ant.

NOT JUST LIKE CLASSIC TANTRA, BUT INSPIRED BY IT

The thing with tantric sex, especially neotantra, is that it does have some of the core tenants that you see in classic tantra, but it's a little bit different. This does acknowledge that most of it is sexual in nature, rather than just focusing on the ancient practices that are there.

Modern tantric sex isn't some weird, obscure thing, but instead, it allows you to be more relevant and meaningful in different ways. There are various ancient practices that are used here, but it incorporates a sense of modernism as well.

THE TANTRA FOCUS

Tantra focuses on their own energies as the main goal of it. The idea behind the tantra is to probe the little parts of life and the energies that are there.

Some people think tantra is associated with or is part of the Vedas. That's not the case, nor did it fully oppose the Vedas either. While it does have some roots in Buddhism and Hinduism, it's in it of its itself its own thing. The reason being is that tantra focuses on the energies, and the relationship of these energies, and the energies both within and without in our lives. The emphasis is on the practice rather than the hypothesis that is there. They oftentimes have the philosophical doctrines in place and will only show them when they need to explain their worldview to others. For the most part, the main idea of tantra is the energies at hand, and what they mean for you.

They are also independent thinkers, and their loyalty was to the truth in it of itself.

Tantra focuses on the concept of energies, and they didn't care as much about the doctrines of every single religious group.

While there is a practice in place, of course, the idea of tantra and tantric sex is something that they can do as a separate action compared to other types of practices.

Intercourse is an aspect of tantra, and tantric texts do talk about it, and the practice of tantra is a more advanced part of the tantric sadhana, and while there are preparatory steps for ritualistic texts, the nice thing about tantra, is that you can prepare yourself in your own way. There are breathing techniques within tantric and tantric sex which are used to help achieve higher spiritual wellness and understanding.

Tantric sex also has different levels of esoterism. Many of these texts have different passages about tantra and tantric sex that discuss this. Many don't realize that while they could be practicing one type of tantra, there are other forms of it, and many people can use it in a ritualistic sense, and the actions at hand.

YOUR ENERGIES ARE THE FOCUS

Tantra and tantric sex are all about your energies and coexisting in a harmonious way. Most don't realize this until they start doing this, but all of us have an energy that's within us, something that keeps us grounded and happy. If we have energies that are in balance, we'll be happy, but if they're somehow not in balance, that causes problems of you now just now, but also in the future too.

Most don't realize the full power of tantra, but with tantric sex, you're experiencing the sexual aspects of it, and the way your energies come together in a way that benefits you.

Tantra involves looking at the liberation of these energies, and liberation in a sexual nature. Most of us don't have sex as a way to feel liberated, but we might. But, with tantric sex, we want as the end-goal to liberate us from our own lives, and to live free in this world.

Most of the people that practice tantra is going for this goal. With other religious doctrines and the like, the goal is to smother this desire. Look at Christianity, where they discuss sex in a way that's not always positive. Tantra wants you to extricate yourself from the burdens of this world, and start to live a life that's more joyful, and full of hope. Many don't realize that all our lives, we live with these bindings in place, and tantric sex works to get out of this.

The idea behind tantra is to have slow, filling movements and soft movements that will help you as a person grow and get even better than ever before. Most don't realize the power of tantra until it's done, and how tantra, when done right, will benefit you immensely in the sexual realm.

Most of us don't feel free in our sexuality. That's because, with the burdens of the world at our disposal, most of us feel constrained by the actions at hand. But, with tantric sex, we can extricate ourselves from those bindings, and in turn, help us bring forth a better, more reliable mission towards one another, and one that will change our lives. We'll be able to face the taboo nature of sex in a more positive manner, and you'll understand that, with each practice of tantric sex, you feel a deeper, more intimate connection with the world.

So, it isn't just freeing your sexual energies between you and your partner, it's also changing the way you approach sex, and the way you handle having sex in the world around you.

Tantric sex allows you to look at yourself in a state where you're most vulnerable, something most of us don't like to do. We don't like to be uncomfortable like this, but with tantric, it's possible. That's because, when we look at ourselves with this type of mindset, we'll realize the power that we have, and how we've held back our energies, but over time, as you start to grow, you'll realize your true power.

Tantra isn't necessarily a ritual in the neotantra sense, but it does involve liberating the body from the bindings, the trauma, and the pain you once felt, bringing forth a better, more rewarding expectation, and to help you bring forth the expectancy that you have. You'll be amazed at the difference life makes when you practice tantra and how, with each passing moment, you'll be able to, with this too, experience the wonders and power of tantric sex, and the fun that this provides.

MEANING OF LOVE AND SEX FOR TANTRA PHILOSOPHY - INTIMACY

So, what is tantric sex at its core? It's pretty in-depth, and here, we'll talk all about what tantric sex is, the concepts behind it, and why it matters.

TANTRIC SEX AT THE CORE

Tantric sex is a type of sexual experience that involves more of slowing down, enjoying what you're doing, and feeling the fun and experience of the moment. It's not quick sex, but more slow, methodical, and fun to experience. The idea behind it is that it's the opposite of a quickie, rushed sex, or anything that seems almost quick and meaningless. This is all about enjoying the other person, and in general, involves increasing intimacy.

The goal of it isn't to just have sex, but it's to experience a deep connection with your partner and is great for serious couples who enjoy it.

AN OLDER PRACTICE

This type of sex isn't just some generic type of sex that you have, but instead, it's a methodical, older process that's important to do. It's an ancient Hindu activity that's been occurring for at least five millennia. So yes, this has been around for a little bit.
The concept behind it is that it's the waving and expansion of different energies, bringing them together in a deep, intimate connection with another being.

It is very slow, and the goal of it is to create a connection between the body and mind. This connection is said to bring about powerful orgasms as a result of it.

It can be done by just about anyone who is physically able to do it. If you want to reboot your sex life, or even find a deeper meaning into the act of making love, this is how you do it.

For most people in this day and age, we all focus on just the action itself, getting it done so we can go about our business. But, does that really build a connection? Are you really focused on your partner? This is what you have to realize happens with tantric sex.

If you are looking for a good way to compare this, a quickie is literally like a takeout food, whereas tantric sex is a five-star meal that you eat in the restraint. With this type of sex, you're not spending as much time just getting it done just to get it done, but it's slow, savoring, and wonderful to experience, and in turn, is a delicious and mesmerizing experience.

This can also bring some space back into your love life. Do you sometimes think you're just having sex just to have sex? Do you sometimes feel like you're not really engaged in the act of sex? Well, that's the problem. For most people, sex is just a quick and dirty thing, rather than an intimate, wholesome action between two parties. That in turn, will cause your relationship to feel hollow, boring, and not worth it.

But, with tantric sex, you can change the way it all feels. Instead of just taking things like an activity and not really putting more emphasis on it than that, tantric sex involves the action of sex, the doingness of it, but also the connection shared between you and the other being you're with.

It's deeper, more thoughtful for both parties, and a ton of fun.

WHY TRY TANTRIC SEX?

There is a reasoning behind trying tantric sex. Tantric sex for one, ash been around for thousands of years. It must work pretty well if you're looking to do something different, and have a deeper, more thoughtful connection with another person.

But, if you want to extend the effort and time into sex, you'll start to get a much more intense ecstasy from it.

Which means a much more intense orgasm.

It does work, and there are even celebrities that will do his with their partners, and it's part of the reason why some people will stay together with one another.

And sometimes, it builds that deep, intimate connection with that person that you want. If you feel like your relationship with your partner is a little stale and boring, this is one of the easiest always to spice things up.

If you're sick of doing the same old, same old in bed, then tantric sex is for you. If you want to become more intimate with the person you love, this is for you. If you would like to reconnect with the one that you love, especially after raising kids, or a stressful day, this is for you.

In the hustle and bustle of our world, we might not think that we have time for this type of sex, but it's a great form of sex, and it can change your life, and the lives of others too.

The concept behind this is where you start to realize that all experience that you have, including sexual intercourse, is a personal thing, and has the potential to transform your ability to understand yourself. Everything in life does this, not just having sex, but we're going to talk about the sexual aspects of this in there.

The idea behind this as well is to be aware and enlightened. You're more aware when you're experiencing tantric sex than you would be if you're just having a quickie with your partner. Perhaps you haven't really looked at your partner all that much recently, or maybe you haven't really thought about anything besides everything you want to do after sex.

Well, tantric sex lets you achieve that awareness of the other person, and it's pretty interesting.

While it does have roots in ancient tantra, it's wonderful for those who want to experience a deeper and more immersive sexual experience.

And what's more, is that tantric sex doesn't involve being spiritual at all. You don't have to be a Hindu to participate in tantric sex, but you can apply these principles in order to have a better life and learn about it as well.

Everything you do during tantric sex is a connection. Whether you both synchronize your breathing together, look a one another, or even touch one another while having intercourse. Unlike other types of sex, it isn't a quick and dirty activity, but instead helps prolong the experience with your partner, and deepen the connection with one another.

DIVINE SEX IN HINDUISM

A great many people follow the way of Tantra to move toward God. God has favored each part of your life; this applies to sex also. You will have the option to interface with God and the heavenly nature, just when you are having intercourse to your partner, since this is the main manner by which you are regarding just as encountering the eternality that dwells inside the human body. The instructing of Tantra immovably expresses that there lies a God in each man and a Goddess in each lady. This infers your body is the vessel for eternality. For accomplishing the critical degrees of shrewdness that are open to you, you will essentially need to relinquish this shell. Your confidence will improve when your partner is regarding you, and you are respecting them consequently. Just when you can see this part of yourself, at exactly that point will you have the option to see the heavenly nature that lives in others also plainly.

Right now, will learn and distinguish the heavenly nature that lives inside you. You will have the option to recognize the God and Goddess inside your body and that of your partner also. This forms the embodiment of Tantric sex. You will likewise have the option to begin to turn out to be progressively edified. This section covers data about various Gods and Goddesses that are famous in Tantric lessons.

THE TERMS 'GOD'
AND 'GODDESS'

As referenced, the lessons of Tantra express that each man and lady ought to be dealt with like a God or a Goddess. This is to ensure that you not just reflect yourself a vessel for eternality however treat your cooperate with a similar see too. Right now, will have the option to regard and respect your partner in the way that you should. This will likewise guarantee that you can respect the force that exists inside the universe.

The various divinities for the most part revered in Tantric sex are viewed as creatures loaded up with light. They symbolize different energies just as connections. Different terms that are generally used for divine beings and goddesses are Deva and Devi, minister and priestess, and Daka and Dakini separately. These gods are accepted to have force and knowledge. This intensity of theirs can likewise be anticipated inside your body. This projection essentially relies upon the different ethics and characteristics that you have.

Goddess is a term that has over and over been used in Tantra. It is used for depicting a lady who is in touch with the ladylike force that dwells inside her body. The underlying significance of this word as a rule implied a lady who was sustaining and solid. A man isn't alluded to as God since God is viewed as a predominant being in different religions. There are a few religions and even a couple of practices that accept that an individual can turn into a divine being or a goddess by changing a couple of parts of themselves. However, the lessons of Tantric sex express that an individual has a specific degree of heavenly nature that is available inside them since birth and there is no hope to change this.

Tantric sex decides express that paying little mind to race, religion or even station of the individual, there's some heavenliness present in everybody. By alluding to a lady as a goddess, you are essentially respecting her female attributes that make her a sweetheart, a tracker, enchantress and supporting person. Just when a lady deals with her attributes and acknowledges herself for what her identity is, will she have the option to respect herself and be regarded by people around her. By tending to a man as a divine being, you are just regarding his essential attributes of being a defender, healer, supplier and an image of intensity. He should acknowledge these qualities that exist inside him and at exactly that point would his be able to partner respect him. You may know about these qualities, or they may just be available inside you, and you haven't found them yet.

DISTINGUISH YOUR JOBS AND ATTRIBUTES

When you are beginning with the excursion towards Tantric sex, then the primary thing that you should do is distinguish the divine beings or the goddesses that characterize you. For doing this, you should recognize your essential attributes and the various jobs that you play in your life. Do you believe yourself to be excellent? It is safe to say that you are keen? It is safe to say that you are a business visionary? It is safe to say that you are amazing? Et cetera. You can record every one of your responses to such inquiries. For making things simpler for yourself, you can make a composition, or you can use mind-mapping too. Place an image of yourself in the focal point of a sheet and afterward begin expounding on all the attributes that you think you have.

When you have accumulated data about the different divine beings and goddesses that has been given in the last piece of this section, you can list down the names of gods that you partner yourself. For example, if you have composed that you are ground-breaking, then maybe you can relate yourself to Shiva or even Ares. If you think you are delightful, then you can record the name of Aphrodite.

LOOK PAST THE SHALLOW LAYER

You presumably will have heard the expression "never pass judgment flippantly." Everyone has likely heard this expression at some point in time. We will in general appointed authority an individual exclusively dependent on their looks, how they dress, or even the activity that they do. You may have offered expressions like "she is excessively thin," or "he is excessively short." You presumably took a gander at an individual's financial balance before consenting to go out on the town with him. In any case, Tantra manages a person's persona and not their shallow attributes. There are three fundamental advances that you should follow to adore the heavenly nature that exists inside your partner.

The initial step is acknowledge that there is eternality that exists inside you. The subsequent advance is to grasp and distinguish the godlikeness that exists inside your partner too. You should find some kind of harmony between the manly and the female energies of the divinities. The third step is join these gods inside you, through your relationship with your partner. This will help in making the genuinely necessary harmony between the two and assist you with achieving a more noteworthy degree of delight.

WHY IS IT IMPERATIVE TO ADORE ONE ANOTHER?

Each individual is more joyful when they realize that they are being recognized. It feels extraordinary when you are valued by the individuals who are around you. Do you know how you feel when somebody sees you? When somebody attempts to get you? Tantric sex is tied in with venerating yourself and your partner too. This doesn't imply that you should adore each other aimlessly. It essentially implies that you both need to shower each other with unequivocal love. Unqualified love doesn't mean genuine control more than each other. It just implies that serving each other as well as could be expected to achieve common joy.

When you begin next the way of Tantric sex, you will find that it feels great to hear positive things about yourself and you will likewise need to continue praising your partner. This is the importance of being revered and venerating your partner.

FINDING OUT ABOUT THE GODS AND GODDESSES

There are diverse male and female divine beings just as goddesses found in various societies around the globe like Egyptian, Greek, Roman and Indian too. These divine beings and goddesses are for the most part from an old time. Let us get familiar with the various goddesses.

The majority of the goddesses frequently sclimax to fruitfulness and life. In any case, they are likewise observed as enchantresses who entice their partners and participate in sex with them. Right now, will find out around a couple of primary goddesses, and you can maybe locate a couple of attributes that you partner yourself with.

Aphrodite:

Aphrodite is viewed as the most acclaimed of Greek goddesses. She sclimaxs to excellence, want, love and sexuality. She additionally sclimaxs to companionship. Aphrodite is regularly spoken to by birds, roses, little dogs and even dolphins too. As indicated by Roman folklore, she is alluded to as Venus. In Roman folklore, she is the image of virtue.

Artemis:

She is viewed as the Goddess of chasing. Artemis is a Greek goddess, and she sclimaxs to the moon and is a virgin goddess. She is a warrior and a tracker, the female partner to supplement Ares, the God of war.

Athena:

The goddess of astuteness and information. She is the supporter goddess of Athens. Technique and arranging are the two attributes that are normally connected with Athena.

Juno:

Juno or Hera, contingent on whether it is the Greek or Roman rendition of folklore is viewed as a mother like figure with a sustaining and a quieting nature.

Hindu Goddesses:

There are different goddesses in India and Nepal, and every one of them has been given a great deal of significance. Different functions are directed to respect each of these goddesses. The fundamental goddesses are referenced here.

Durga is viewed as the mother all things reflected. Tara is reflected to sclimax to astuteness just as graciousness. Lakshmi is the goddess of riches and thriving. Saraswati is the goddess of different works of art and ability. Kali sclimaxs to quality and force. She is likewise the defender of the domain.

DIVINE BEINGS FROM DIFFERENT CULTURES

Each religion has various divine beings and goddesses. These divine beings frequently have a partner as a goddess. There are various divinities loved by various societies. They all sclimax to gigantic quality, force, and are frequently thought of as super creatures. This segment covers carious divine beings from various religions. You may have the option to distinguish your qualities or those of your partner right now here.

Hindu Gods:

Hindu divine beings incorporate Lord Shiva who has gigantic force and Lord Vishnu is viewed as the God all things reflected. There are various indications of Lord Shiva, and there are many portrayals of his clouded side also. Shakti is the associate of Lord Shiva. Master Shiva and Shakti form a ground-breaking match and sclimax to pure energy. Ganesh is a famous god also; he is a little youngster with the leader of an elephant. Master Ganesh is known to expel deterrents and spread satisfaction. Master Rama and Sita form a couple that is frequently loved all over India, they are viewed as the ideal couple and sclimax to the concordance that should exist between a husband and spouse.

Greek divine beings:

There are various Greek divine beings, and they have all become well known in view of the quality and force that they hold. Zeus is viewed as the best of all; he is the King everything being equal and the remarkably ground-breaking Alpha-male. Eros is normally alluded to, as Cupid, and he is seraph or a young man who is regularly fiendish and frequently continues shooting bolts of love at individuals around him. He is the God of love. Dionysus is the Greek and the Roman divine force of desire. As indicated by the legends, he generally pursued ladies and enjoyed drinking a great deal of wine. He for sure is the divine force of desire.

ADVANTAGES AND DIFFERENCES WITH TRADITIONAL SEX

T antric sex and our regular "sexual" sex is very different, and in some ways, people don't even realize the impact of tantric sex, and how it can change the way you have sex.

A DIFFERENT PATHWAY

Regular sex has three different stages: foreplay, the act of intercourse, and of course the climax or ending. Once that's done, it actually is the end, and usually, you're done. Sometimes you have sex and you go back to your normal life.

But tantric sex is different. Tantric sex has zero linear progression. You might not even have an orgasm until after foreplay and intercourse, or maybe even just foreplay brings you to that level. The idea behind it isn't to just focus on the orgasm, and don't use the orgasm as the ending point. It takes away that idea and makes it so that you're not as hung up on it.

THE ENERGIES
THAT ARE THERE

The energy that's in a regular bout of sex is different. It's purely sexual, penis or vagina against another genitalia, and the whole act is physical. Whether it be kissing, rubbing, pinching, or even penetration he idea behind it is physical, and not as mental. Oftentimes, people might not even look at one another, and it is something that you need to realize makes tantric sex a little different.

The connection that's there during tantric sex isn't just a physical manifestation, but it's also a different type of manifestation of energy. This is more than just sexual energy, but they try to expand that energy from the genitalia out to the rest of the body, so it can cause pleasure in different forms. The pleasure and energies that are there are actually not just the actions of the movements of the body, but the way your partner feels, and the mental energy that's there. It allows you to have a deeper feeling with this, and it is a much more intimate activity tan just regular sex in most cases.

WORKING TOGETHER

The thing with regular sex is, usually the endgame of it is an orgasm, to have that release, and then you're done. You're more focused on that than just working and experiencing the moment together.
The crazy thing about tantric sex is you can have an orgasm not just from the act of intercourse alone. Some people have an orgasm from massages, from light foreplay, even pinching or biting the nipples can result in a tantric orgasm. The idea of it is to stop worrying so much about orgasms, and instead, focus on the moment.

You want to make sure that your breathing is similar to your partner's, and it isn't out of sorts, and it isn't labored or wavering. You also want to keep eye contact with one another.

This is something that most people don't realize they don't do when they engage in regular sex. Whether it be doggy-style or even just turning the lights off instead of on, people are scared to look at one another. Maybe it's the vulnerability of the moment, but it actually can change the way it makes you feel. Tantric sex brings you out of the "only me" mindset during sex, making you more selfless, and helping you attain that connection over time.

TIME SPENT

The time spent during sex usually varies, but most people usually don't spend more than an hour together in the bedroom, unless of course, they want to go long. Sometimes, the quickie sessions last all but five minutes, and that's it. But, here's the thing, tantric sex can last a long time, several hours at that.

That's partially because they aren't trying to do this just to get off, but instead, they want to submerge into a way where they can cyclically go together and experience intercourse. The crazy thing about this is that tantric sex causes more orgasms and more powerful orgasms than standard sex does.

The end of the game isn't a depletion of the physical energies, but instead, you're both experiencing a cyclical direction of you both experiencing the fun and pleasure of one another, and the pleasure and intensity spent.

THE TOUCHING

The limitation of regular sex is that it focuses mostly on physical touch and it doesn't work on a higher plane than that. But, the crazy thing about tantric sex, is that they may not touch one another in some cases. Sometimes, people might just barely move their hands there, and sometimes, they feel an increased series of pleasure.

It also causes orgasm waves as well. This is because tantric sex isn't just a small little wave of pleasure, but instead a deeper, almost mesmerizing wave of pleasure that comes from the orgasm that's there too. It's amazing how this can change the way that you feel, and the pleasure and fire that goes through this.

Tantric sex doesn't always involve a bunch of touching, nor does it have to involve extreme pain or anything that's here. Instead, it can be a wave of orgasms that are different, and powerful as well.

The wild thing about tantric sex is that it involves a pure and mesmerizing form of energy with one another, and it helps to develop and broaden your ability to experience pleasure.

THE STRONGEST ENERGY

Some people think tantric sex isn't the strongest form of energy, but it is. That's because it's a human connection directly through energy, and with physical sex, sure you're touching, but sometimes the full-on connection isn't like that. Tantric sex is to regular sex what yoga is to your average gym workout. Both are great, but the thing is, if you want a deeper connection physically and mentally with your partner, you oftentimes will feel it within the body through tantric sex, rather than just through your average bout in the bedroom. Tantric sex spreads through the entire body, and it permeates through, almost like a sponge soaking up all of that energy and then releasing it outwards.

Tantric sex is a way for you to manifest the spirit, and in some ways, that's why people argue that tantric sex is the most powerful form of sex, because it involves the spirit, through the action of making love. It's a form of intimacy that's very valid and has many different principles that are incredibly valid, and worth mentioning.

Tantric sex is the better form of sex for that reason alone. It promotes a deeper, more worthwhile connection with the person you love.

With tantric sex, you can actually get closer and closer to divinity, and you can experience the masterpiece of it. It's a more spiritual, more rewarding and close sex that allows you to experience the divinity. Tantric sex is a wonderful way to really bring you closer to your partner.

STIMULATES A BETTER RELATIONSHIP

People don't realize that just because you have sex doesn't mean it's meaningful to your partner. Sometimes, you have sex to get off, or to experience pleasure, but you don't really experience the fun and deep connection of a relationship with your partner if you're just having regular sex.

Sure, regular sex is fun for some people, and it can bring about a deep, rewarding connection, but the problem is, oftentimes it creates a bit of a hollow relationship with your partner. Some people just have sex to keep the relationship going, but tantric sex isn't about that.

Not all sex is done with the idea of building a connection in mind. Sometimes it's done to just orgasm and that's it. But tantric sex lets you foster a better, deeper connection with your partner, and allows you to have empowered sexuality via arousal and stimulating the senses. You start to experience a comeback of the deepen erotic nature of the senses of sex, and many people realize it creates a more aligned, meaningful experience with your partner.

Many people love this form of sex because it helps bring a more meaningful way to love another human being. Humans want to show to their partner how much they love them, and the thing with tantra is that allows you to really feel the romance, and really spice things up.

You want to bring new things to the table, and tantric sex lets you do that.

Romance isn't dead, it's just you get hung up by routines. Tantra is a way for you to keep sex alive and well in your life. And you don't even need to believe in antra to do it. If you want to practice the positions and the fun of it, then you can easily do so through the power of sex.

For most people, the don't realize how their relationship has changed, and they might not realize they even pay attention to your partners. But, with tantric sex, you'll be able to really foster a better, deeper connection with the person that you love, and bring forth a better, more reliable connection with yourself, and with your partner as well.

IS TANTRIC SEX BETTER?

Now that's not to say you shouldn't ever have regular sex again. You should have sex how you want to have sex, but you should understand that tantric sex stimulates your entire body and forces you to move into a state of vulnerability and wellness. For many people, tantric sex depends on the connection and the love that you share with your partner. If you've ever been curious about tantric sex, it can only help you.

But, the thing with tantric sex, is that it's very long.it takes a long time since there is no end goal. If you want to have normal sex with your partner, then go for it, but understand that it may not have as deep of a connection.

Does tantric sex save relationships? Perhaps, but also understand that sex won't fix everything about a relationship, and if it's already a sinking ship, then you may want to figure out other alternatives and means to really help you get the most out of your sexual relationship. For many, tantric sex builds it all, and makes it so that you're able to build and foster that connection with people that you love. The one that you love matters a lot, and that's why many people enjoy the fun of tantric. It's because, it isn't just the sex act itself, but also the act of being connected with the person around you, and the one that you love.

Now that you understand that, you'll see how tantra betters the full spirit, whereas regular sex I mostly a physical affair. Both are wonderful to experience, but if you feel like fostering a deeper, more meaningful connection with the person that you love, tantra is the name of the game and its key for that.

That's why many people love tantra because it allows for you to foster that love and understanding with the one that you're with. It can improve your health, wellness, and happiness too.

So, which is best? The answer is tantra, but it's also important to understand the differences. Both of them do have their pros and cons, and you'll understand that, with each moment and each experience you share with your partner, there are a lot of benefits to be had with this and a lot that you certainly should try to enjoy.

HOW BEST TO PREPARE YOUR MIND AND BODY FOR TANTRIC SEX USING TECHNIQUES FOR FOREPLAY, MASSAGE, AND MASTURBATION

TALK TO YOUR PARTNER

Before you begin with this, always make sure that you and your partner both want to try this. Remember, it takes two to tango, and that goes for tantric sex especially. If you're interested in doing it, you need to make sure that your partner is on the same page as you are. Most people don't realize that this is something that your partner may not be ready for.
While you think starting right away is a great idea, but here's the thing: you have to, with tantric sex, discuss this since it is a two-part procedure and something that you'll have to do together. If you're both not interested or working together, it won't happen.

Plus, if you're practicing tantric sex but they're not, it would mean only one of you is going to experience powerful orgasms and want to take it slower, while the other will be doing the opposite. It seems a little bit unfair, right? That's the main issue you run into with tantric sex if you experience it any other way, it's that you're not going to make it work, and you won't really get the results.

And it shouldn't be hard to convince your partner to try it. After all, you want deeper intimacy between you and the other person, better sex, more passion, and just more fun between the two of you.

This is simple to get your partner's agreement on since it is probably something, they'll enjoy from the spicing up and variety alone.

PREPARE THE BODY

Preparing the body is a good thing to do with tantric sex because it takes time. Oftentimes, people don't realize that tantric evenings can be a bit physically demanding. It oftentimes also makes you feel better about yourself too. You'll appreciate the way your body feels, and the wellness you experience.
When you feel good physically and the room is arranged how it should be, it'll tranquilize you, making lovemaking some of the best there is.

So what are some things that you can do? Well first and foremost, if you're not someone who wants to spend hours at the gym, or work too hard on their physical fitness, then try yoga.

Yoga is one of the best choices that you'll experience. It is a great thing that will help with improving your experience.

Not only that, yoga helps with flexibility, and there are postures that will change your sex life too. Some of them can even be used during tantric sex. Plus, it helps with realigning the energy.

It's deduced that energies you have flowed from your spine, so you should always make sure that you have a relaxed back that isn't hunched over. You should also do this n a way where you're not hurting yourself, and it isn't physically affecting the back.

DIET TIPS

Diet is the next area to focus on. Diet is actually on par with physical fitness, but for tantric nights it also helps improve them. Diet doesn't mean you have to follow a complex menu that some guru put together, but what you should do is eat in a manner that's healthier than ever. The best way to do it is to have habits that are healthy, and you practice moderation. Try to abstain from overindulging as you get closer and closer to the tantric night. You should try to not eat a lot of heavier foods right before having tantric sex, and also don't overconsume alcohol either.

You should stay hydrated, but also not drink a ton of water too much once you get closer to time. That's because you want to keep things steamy, and while bathroom breaks happen, you don't want that hindering everything.

Also, look for safe detox recipes, with the focus being on safe. You should look for ones that have happy users, and those who have some complaints so you could also look at the difference between them.

Don't look for reviews that are overly happy either. That's because, happy reviews are faked, but the negative ones aren't either. But you should also look at safety concerns too. If you have a condition that's also affecting your ability to do a diet, also research the side effects of that.

You should also try to snack minimally, and if you do snack, you should also be mindful of what you're eating. There's a lot that you can eat that's healthy and good for you, and a lot that you should minimize. Go through and look for all of these, so you can better understand what you're doing, and also don't overindulge in these as well. Because let's face it, do you really need to gorge on those cookies? Probably not.

RELAXING THE BODY

Before you get into tantric sex, you should try to relax the body. Relaxing the body is very important because if you're not relaxed, you're going to feel a bit exhausted, and probably sick from the stress. After a bad day, even if you didn't do a whole lot, it'll feel like you've fought with a bear and lost.
The body is important to relax, but you should also make sure that you relax the mind to. Mental stress does weaken your immune system, and bacteria and viruses love when that happens.

Learning to relax is a possible thing, but the big thing to remember here is to not float around like you're in a Zen haze. You might live in a chronic-stress situation though, and that becomes the new normal for many. Lots of times, people don't realize how stressed out they are, and the debts, demands, and coping skills oftentimes are a reason why people drift apart. This is a big thing to understand because tantra helps you build a bond that's closer than ever before, that's more than just sex for many people.

Oftentimes, relaxing is a hard-pressed concept. You probably might have issues with a long-term stress reliever, but a nap, a shower, or a movie that's funny is definitely helpful. Meditation is valuable, but it's an overlooked thing, but you need to learn to accept that you're stressed out, and you need to spend time preparing yourself for this. If you're a bit sad about the way that you look, try to maybe spend 30 minutes a day walking or working out. It does bring about liberation to you in its own way. Plus, if you're relaxed, you'll practice tantra way better, and accept all of this in the long run.

WHAT TO WEAR

Some people think that you need to wear very tight and sexy clothes. No, wear something that's loose, comfortable, and you should try to put something on that makes you feel good. Some people will dress in attire that reflects certain deities or the east. But it can help bring about the art of tantra into the bedroom. However, you should also focus on being clean and happy with yourself before you practice tantra. First, brush your teeth and hair prior to what you do. This is a quick and simple thing to really bolster your confidence and make it easier for you to do as well.

Some people like to do a ritual bath beforehand, but that is something that you don't have to do. You should make sure that it's a bit structured, and that you have the aim of making sure that you are bonded, but not bonded enough to have sex yet. You should wash one another in ways that are on-sexual and use soaps and oils that are scented. This fosters anticipation between the two people, and it's something that you'll enjoy with the other person.

You should do things together that foster anticipation between both of you as well. That will, in turn, benefit both of you, and it does bring about an honorable and artful experience with your partner.

SETTING YOUR SCENE

You should set the scene up by putting rituals into sex, and make sure that your space is set up. Most people focus on making sure there's a lot of white in the room, such as in the form of pillows, candles, and also soft music. You should do this with the intent of making the sex feel special.

For most people, they just rush into the bedroom and don't really work to set the mood. But, if you really want to make it memorable for both parties, you should try decorating it. Soft, sensual music will help bring forth a better, more intimate experience between both of you. Music is great for sex period, but soft, sensual music will change the way sex is for both parties and brings forth a sense of understanding, wellness, and happiness as well.

BREATHE AWAY!

Before you even start, you should breathe and make sure that you do it in a way that benefits you. This is a good way to mentally calm yourself down, and to help you relax. What you should do, is take one full breath in through the nose, fill the belly with air, and then exhale. You should notice your belly move outwards. That's your diaphragm breathing, and you should make sure that you do focus on getting that type of breathing. When you exhale, you should see the belly start to return to normal size.

If you're having issues with this, you should visualize that pushing the pelvis down through there, and you push the breath directly to the floor. Try to do this a few times before you do it during sex so it becomes more automatic so that you can really benefit from this too.

TRY MASSAGES

Finally, before you have sex, you should try massaging. These massages don't have to be a long time, but you should try to switch off between the giver, and the receiver of leisure. You might ask your partner to rub your feet for a couple of minutes, and then do whatever they like for a couple of minutes.

During each turn, don't be afraid to give the feedback that you need to. It's okay to tell your partner what it is they should do better, and this will help them really give you what you want.

This is something most couples struggle with. By talking to the other person, you will be able to really get what you want. Communication is something that most people need to understand has to be there. The way you work together is a great way for you to learn. You will be able to teach your lover what you want, and they'll teach you what they want, creating the best sexual experience possible for you.

You should pay attention to the way their hands feel, the way they touch you, the sensual nature of this, and from there, relax the body and the mind. This will help you improve your ability to handle this, and make it so that you're happier and better than ever.

TANTRA EXERCISES AND MASSAGES FOR SEXUAL FULFILLMENT OF COUPLES

Originating in what is now modern India; Tantra is at least 5000-7000 or more years old, pre-dating and influencing both Hinduism and Buddhism.

Many religions believe you can have either physical pleasure or spiritual growth, but not both.

Tantra flatly disagrees, believing that physical and sensual pleasure are themselves the key to our spiritual growth; without one, you can't have the other.

Tantrics believe working on our bodies can clear them of accumulated rubbish, enabling healing and re-integration with the surrounding spirit energy. Central to Tantra is its belief in this spirit or energy force, and that the universe - and us individually - are all filled with the same energy. Crucially, Tantrics believe that any repression of this energy leaves us unbalanced and damaged.

Tantra rejects the repressive, moralistic, self-denying code of living propounded by many religions, where our body's sexual or sensual needs are met with guilt, more guilt, repression, denial and punishment. Where, when attention is paid to bodily needs, it's usually aimed at avoidance, for example of disease or pregnancy. Little attention is paid to the development and expansion of our body's sensuality; no teaching us how to embrace it, value it.

Tantrics believe that to grow as complete beings, blockages need clearing from both our physical and psychic systems. Most people accept the idea of physical systems. We all know we have a Liver, Heart, and Stomach for example - but psychic systems? Controversial - but nevertheless, most major religions, do believe that we are more than our physical body.

Tantrics believe that a powerful spirit energy, lives in our Base Chakra, situated between our legs. Once released, it rises through our system. If dormant, our knowledge is limited; aroused it allows the natural spiritual growth we should be experiencing.

This vital energy- Kundalini - is 'fed' along channels called Meridians. Any obstruction lessens energy flow, much as a kinked hose-pipe produces only a reduced water supply.

Many believe that one manifestation of the 'Life Energy' is the Aura. Whether it is actually an aura, with its quasi-religious overtones or 'only' electricity' is, hotly debated. Some recent scientific research however confirms a generalised electromagnetic current around our body and that all tissue and each individual organ, such as the Heart and the Brain also generates an individual impulse. Is there a link between this comparatively recent research and the Tantric belief in the Chakra system - spinning wheels of energy, spiralling throughout our body, where the various aspects and levels of our 'being' are merged? When these energy centres function properly, Tantrics believe, so do we. As with the Meridians, however, factors such as lifestyle, conditioning, guilt, diet, prevent them from fully functioning. Once they're 'clogged' we become sluggish, under-performing.

Tantrics, and some modern therapies, believe we have many such blockages and that trauma, such as remembered grief, pain, embarrassment, physical or emotional abuse, remains stored in our body. The effects of this early blocking continue throughout our life, reducing our well-being, our energy; we may, perhaps, constrict our throats because of childhood conditioning to 'don't cry,' or 'don't shout'. Our pelvis may be rigid through our attempts to stifle our genital urges. Our anal sphincter may have tightened, and remain tight as the result of our early - and long forgotten- attempts to repress anger.

THE MASSAGE

Believing our body is utterly central to our well-being; Tantrics use many techniques to 'repair' it. One such is massage, it's believed that massage and Tantric techniques can help break down blockages and flush them out, - that the massage can heal us.

Tantric massage uses many techniques familiar in other massages, so what differentiates it from other forms of massage?

I would suggest five things;

1. Therapeutic masseurs focus on direct physical benefits; sensualists see pleasure as an end in itself. Tantrics go further, believing that the pleasure is the gateway to spirituality - the means to an end.

2. In Tantra we give without seeking a return; receive without feeling we have to reciprocate.

3. It is a way of giving and receiving sensual pleasure without needing to perform in any sexual way.

4. No externally imposed barriers exist as to where, what and how to touch. The only barriers are those that we, as responsible adults have decided will be there. If the agreement allows exploration of the whole of your partner's body, they -and you -may find new, totally unexpected, areas of enjoyment. Many

Westerners tend to be very genitally orientated. We overlook the other 95% of our body, much of which is capable of giving differing but equally exquisite responses. In this way, Tantra continues the liberation many feel when they realise that touch is both natural and mutually enriching.

5. There are techniques for both breathing and massaging particular areas of the body, such as the Chakras or genitals that are specific to Tantra, or the Chinese Tao.

Tantra is a letting go, a sensual journey that can lead to astounding joy. Striving to be open and honest, it is an uplifting but disciplined approach to the body. It permits - encourages - a freedom to experience, experiment, enjoy and openly delight in our body in a way that we in the West can find in turns, alarming, exhilarating, shaming and - perhaps - ultimately liberating. The results of this openness, allied to it's emphasis on the journey not the destination being important can be astounding for those used to concentrating on the journey's end (i.e. ejaculation for the man which it discourages, and, if she's lucky, orgasm for the woman). It allows time for us to focus on our partner and their body's varied sensations. Tantra has, few, if any, taboos, provided -and it is a big proviso - that whatever is done is done with mutual respect and unforced agreement. Power, coercion, emotional blackmail or exploitation is not acceptable in Tantra...

For all the above reasons Tantra is ideally suited to a massage

SENSUAL MALE MASSAGE TECHNIQUE

For centuries, Tantric sex and massage has been a way not only to get nearer to each other, but to also help you develop a deep connection with your other half, yourself and the world around you. Through Tantric massage or male erotic massage, you can discover the benefits of being with a partner you love, who understands the fundamentals of male genital massage. There's a standard parable that Tantric massage is a sexual massage, and while there is a sexual facet to it, it is more about healing yourself and lover through self-discovery and the use of sexual energy.

Tantric massage is a divine experience that is related to the non secular factors of the Tantra. Truly, the word Tantra means 'personal growth in a pleasurable existence'. Through this massage, you can begin to experience pleasure like you never thought possible and since it is Tantric, it is highly non secular and something that will leave you awakened to the cosmos, yourself and everything around you. There are multiple strategies to perform Tantric male massage, but regularly it involves the calm motions of the hand along the head and shaft of the penis to extend the pleasure of the experience for the masseuse and the individual receiving the erotic male massage. Through the course of the massage, a stress on peaceful, fingertip touching must be kept to make certain the correct experience is achieved through the Tantric massage.

It is important to remember the point isn't sex with Tantric massage, but to meet an intensely intense experience between you and your other half. We debated earlier that there are benefits to sex, and while Tantric massage isn't sex, it is based in sexual energy and the use of sexual energy has enormous benefits to the body.

Whether it is through the method of healing of sexual energy, or through the silence and stress reduction that comes from Tantric massage. The fantastic thing about Tantric male massage isn't that it feels good, but that it's got many health and stress reduction benefits not only for the person receiving the massage, but for the person giving the massage too.

Both folks will be ready to use this out of the ordinary intimate experience where both will become close through the technique of discovering their partner and discovering themselves.

By massaging the penis of the individual and helping them awaken to new realms of pleasure, the masseuse helps to raise the individual's mind to a new realm which will help them become calm, picked up and better prepared to manage life around them. It is important to understand the benefits of Tantric male massage, but not to confuse it with sex. Sexual energy is some of it, but the physical act of Tantric massage isn't sex, it is self discovery with someone you love. If you are considering performing Tantric massage on someone, then you are opening up a totally new world to them, helping them discover things about themselves and you, through the use of Tantric male massage.

HOT MASSAGE TIPS - TANTRIC MASSAGE

ot Massage Tips: Tantric Massage

Before we discuss this type of massage in more detail, we need to understand that Tantric massage is unique and a very special kind of massage. As with other forms of massage, Tantric massage has its own unique benefits. What particularly appeals to me is how this focuses more on our feelings and spiritual well being rather than our physical health.

Unfortunately, it's not that common and, therefore, not readily available just everywhere due to the specialist skills and training involved. The professional who provides such massage services must be a master of the basic and advanced principles of Tantra and meditation.

The Tantric massage experience always begins with ancient Tantric rituals and a time of meditation in order to focus on the Chakras and the spiritual link with the entire universe.

You must always keep in mind that this kind of massage is not meant to relieve the stresses and strains that our bodies have been subjected to, to work the muscles, or to focus on our physical well being. Tantric massage awakens the hidden mystic energy and brings your body and spirit in complete harmony with the universe.

Tantric massage makes use of light, sensual and slow strokes that can channel energy and increase the body's sensitivity to a different reality. You may wish to apply some medium pressure along the sides of the spine in order to make your massage effective, but otherwise confine yourself to light pressure and to the movements inspired from the way energy flows through the body and especially the classic movement upwards from the base of the spine.

 I would suggest that this form of massage should not be taken lightly. Don't play at it. A great deal of skill is required as well as an in-depth knowledge of your inner energy before even contemplating conducting a Tantric massage.

I am sure the values and benefits of a Tantric massage have been undermined because people may well have "tried it" without understanding its true meaning and the highly specialized skills required to perform a true Tantric massage.

Meditation and music are the only things you need for this kind of massage. However, the music used should be known for its connections with meditation and spiritual awareness. There is music designated for use with Tantric massage but it is not commonplace and may be hard to find.

Although unnecessary, oils and lotions can also be used and, I suppose there may be a perception that a massage would not be a massage without them. So as not to diminish the overall effect of this type of massage, avoid the use of scented oils as they can, in themselves, be distracting.

Try Tantric massage with your partner. When performed successfully, it undoubtedly increases your levels of intimacy and develops a stronger emotional and spiritual bond between the two of you.

This is achieved by building on the love and trust that exists instead of focusing on sex.

MASSAGE TECHNIQUES

Tantra has much more meaning than what we understand. Its origins are in India and date back over 5000 years ago. Without using a lot of words, tantra focuses on energy, sensual energy distribution across the body and not so much the mind. It teaches us how to open our hearts and our sexuality. In tantra, sex is like a game of football with team managers and the technical bench taking notes and punctuating the players as the game goes on. Tantra is that rich it has professional teachers, counselors and trainers.

When beginning a massage, your partner, referred to as the receiver lies flat with support of pillows or any other material, while to giver takes control of the task. The stuck naked body lying down on a bed with fully exposed genitals is supposed to begin with deep relaxed breathing. This breathing is a switch towards achieving full relaxation and it has to be done at intervals while massage is going on. Massage oil is used and as it moves on, constant reminding must be done for the receiver to breath deep.

For a man, the entire male organ, scrotum, pubic bone, g-spot, testicles, perineum etc are the target areas to work on. Massage the whole body to get him relax fully and cool down, then proceed to the penis and hold onto it firmly. Lift like you want to pluck it so as to massage the testicles gently; move the shaft side ways, left, forward like a gear handle of an automobile. Take time speed is not part of the exercise; feelings and the radiation of energy is the in thing. Massage the head to tune the nerves and get a healing in return; if incase ejaculation is tempted, back off and touch other areas. Reach the g-spot if you can so as to expand his orgasm and fix his inability to control ejaculation. At this area be gentle and soften it more because at first it is often uncomfortable.

In case of a woman being the receiver, start with the exposed breast; take your time as she breaths deeply. Breast are great assets, feel the radiation of love from them, move around them gently; then extend to the belly. Proceed to the pubic zone and avoid the vulva area incase she might get aroused. Massage her fully up to the toes and monitor how she behaves. Find out her readiness; sexual energy distribution is important and its distribution is life itself. The raised spirits makes tantric very elaborate and enjoyable.

Tantric sex is very detailed and enjoyable; it makes men stay longer in the act, even for a whole night, while women get restoration of full orgasm and satisfaction. It is not a few minutes spiking and snoring thereafter, love making is a process, and it goes through its turns bringing entire relief with your partner. Link love with sexual pleasure as it overflows from your heart; concentrate, feel the stimulation as you gaze at one another for a while. When ready let the organs meet and hold one another and feel the intense energy flowing across the body up to the head. Remain focused and taste the pleasure of the genitals meeting point, don't accelerate into anything; sex is all about being fully charged and remaining still.

HOW TO EXPERIENCE A GREAT TANTRA MASSAGE

There are various ways to learn and practice Tantra. Among all the ways, tantric massage is the most resulting one. A good tantra massage includes several other components than only the massage. Proper meditation, tantric yoga, breathing, relaxation, and effective sexual techniques are the other components of such a massage.

A tantra massage, unlike other massage techniques, requires an emotional bonding between the giver and the receiver. It is quite natural that a stranger cannot satisfy a person in any way like a familiar person can do. Therefore, it is a good idea to avoid all the commercials that claim to give effective tantric massage. Proper trust and proper intimacy are the two basic things of various tantra rituals, exercises, and tantra techniques.

A person requires should do certain things for a good tantra massage. First of all, the massage should take place in such an environment that is useful to offer complete relaxation of both body and mind. The place should also be free from any kind of disturbances. The place better be detached from any kind of contact with the outside world.

The surface on which the massage would take place is equally important like the environment. Since comfort and relaxation are the most sought after things, a soft mattress, mat, or even a fresh sheet can do the work. Towels offering proper support to the knees and neck area are must. Avail great quality massage oil made of herbs, which can enhance the effectiveness of the massage. There are certain other things which can boost the level of relaxation attained through tantric massage. Mild incense, soft pious music, and candlelight can definitely do the magic.

The receiver should recline on his her stomach as the massage starts. A gentle foot massage is the ideal thing to start the massage. Gradually, the treatment should shift towards the neck and shoulder area. The important pressure points those are present in the neck and shoulder area can offer best relaxation throughout the body if treated with proper massage strokes. The back area is the next place where the masseur should focus on. The joints and the muscular areas should receive proper care to help the receiver get rid of all the stress. When the back area is complete, the receiver should slowly turn around. This will help the masseur take care of the front area.

EMOTIONAL AND CULTURAL CONSENT: WHAT IT IS AND WHY IT MATTERS

Tantric sex does require you to have consent, just like all forms of sex. But, it's a little different this time around.

CONSENT: WHY IT'S SEXY

For most people, consent is something that should always be there, but it's something that not only allows for sexual situations to be a mutually-beneficial activity, but it's also the difference in many cases between sex and of course, rape and abuse.

Consent is something that you should always work towards having. Most people don't understand the impact nonconsensual activities are on someone, whether it be sex or otherwise, and consent allows for you to subject yourself to this, so you're happier and healthier.

But consent isn't just in a physical consent. The whole "I'm okay with you touching me there" is impactful, but it's more than just a physical action.

It's also, an emotional, mental and cultural type of agreement.

Physical consent is usually given in most relationships. You say it's okay to have sex, and then you do it. But tantric sex requires emotional and cultural consent, and both of these are something that usually most sex doesn't have. Sex can be emotional, but usually, you don't need heavy emotional consent when you're having sex. But, with tantra, it is a very emotional activity, and you need to understand that, in order to have a successful tantra experience, you must give the consent to experience the emotions of yourself, and of other people.

WHAT IS EMOTIONAL CONSENT

Emotional consent is where you consent to the emotions that someone else either gives to you, or you provide.

Have you ever talked to someone where, at first, it's just you talking about your problem, but your friend suddenly jumps forward, giving unsolicited advice on how to handle the situation? Have you ever done this? Oftentimes, emotional consent is just as important as physical consent. It isn't good to be on either side of those types of interactions, and for most people, jumping into that oftentimes means that your conversations will be disappointing, and it can oftentimes be very frustrating to deal with.

The problem is that we live in a world that's messy, and you need to understand that you have to build deeper connections with other people that you come into contact with. But the thing is, you need to give the okay to experience those types of emotions. To do otherwise allows you to build trust with the other person, and it leaves you both a place to share your thoughts.

Talking to others is tiring. Emotional labor is something that most of us don't sign up for, and emotional consent is very important because it honors the ability to give the other person the perspective that you have, and also, so that they're not being bombarded with these emotions and instead, you both set healthy, happy boundaries with others.

Emotional consent is as simple as you're both okay with feeling the effects of it, and also how you can benefit from this as well.

Emotional consent is more than just "I'm willing to listen to your problems" though. Lots of times, emotional consent in tantra is allowing yourself to be exposed to some of the harsher realities of the world.

When you experience tantra, you go through a lot of emotions, and oftentimes, you both have to be on the same page. Breathing together, looking at one another, experiencing the flow of one another's energies can be tough, especially after a long day. That's why, if you practice tantric sex it's important to do this when you're not hung up on the distractions of life and instead, you're able to easily understand and utilize the information that you learn about your partner.

It's a very spiritual activity, and you need to consent to get into those kinds of emotions. Sometimes, when you do this too, you tackle traumatic points.

TACKLING TRAUMA AND EMOTIONAL CONSENT

The emotions you experience during tantric sex aren't just the emotions of yourself and the other person. Tantric sex is done to free yourself from the bindings of other people, and oftentimes, what people don't realize is, that with tantric sex it can be a very stimulating process for both parties.

Tantric sex involves looking at the traumatic associations with sex too. For many of us, we don't spend time enjoying the moment, and the emotions associated with this. But, with tantric sex, we can overcome the problems of the past, and from there, face the future. However, you need to understand that it is an emotionally-stimulating thing and it can be good for you, but also very heavy. Understand that you're also opening yourself up to the trauma and problems that your partner faces too, which is why many people don't realize the full power of tantric sex. For most of us tantric sex helps us understand our own personal wellness and ability to really explore the unknown.

Consenting to this is important, consent is something that you need to have emotionally and sexually during tantric sex, but you need to understand that you must freely give consent, are giving informed consent, are enthusiastic about I, and you communicate with the other person what's going on.

Communicating especially during the more traumatic elements might be good for you. It lets you explore these desires, and these feelings in a healthy way. Remember, you're also looking at sexual boundaries, eliminating them and being free, which will, in turn, help you with improving your own wellness and happiness. Consent is really good not just for looking at the emotional aspects of I, but also to handle trauma related to this subject, which is more common than you think.

CONSENT AS A CULTURE

Tantric sex encourages you to fully consent to everything that you do. That's the culture of it. When you engage in tantra, the goal of it is liberation, and you need to agree to the idea that, with tantra, you're going to experience new things related to it, and it can be a big thing for most people.

You need to understand that you should speak up for yourself, and your own personal feelings. You shouldn't just blindly follow what the doctrines teach you, or if you're doing it with someone know knows tantra, also work to form your own conclusions as well. You should stay within your comfort zones in relation to tantra in order to minimize any changes of later regrets.

Always state your boundaries during tantric sex. If you like the massaging feeling of being touched in some areas, but not in other areas, you should always make sure you let the person know that you're with.

You should understand as well that you should never do group coercion either. Never just feel like you need to do something because it's said. Some people are definitely better by discussing things, and the culture of tantra encourages you to discuss this with the other person, so both of you are on the same page, and are honest with one another.

When doing tantra, always make sure to have honest feedback in place when doing this. If there are some things that you didn't like, let your partner know, and some things that you do like, again, let them know as well. You should always practice mutual consent with your partner, and make sure that you're both on the same page.

And as always, understand that tantra is a very personal thing. You don't need to scream to everyone about what happened during your five-hour tantric sex experience. That's something that should only be discussed between both of you, and not something that you should just keep out in the open. Keep the confidentiality of it in place, because it'll help with improving the sexual experience, and the wellness you share as well.

BOUNDARIES STILL MATTER IN TANTRA

Finally, remember your boundaries in tantric sex is still a big thing here. That's because, even though tantric sex involves going with the flow and doing things that stimulate your mind along with the body, you have to understand that there are still some boundaries that you shouldn't cross.

If that ever gets violated, that's not okay. That's assault, and that's something that you should never have happen. Instead, be honest with your partner, and you should also make sure that boundaries are discussed in a way that's fitting for everyone, and in a way that's safe.

As always, just like with any other type of sexual experience, tis very important you keep your consent in place, and you try to work on being consensual, and also willing to work together. You should try to as well, make sure that you understand the value of consent, and what happens when you consent with your partner. Discuss this early on, but always make sure that you do have these worked out, both physically and emotionally, and the type of cultural consent you'll have.

Cultural consent can be something as simple as tying a ritualistic experience with it or wearing similar clothing to signify it. Always talk with your partner before you begin with this, and make sure you're both on the same page regarding it, because that alone will help improve your experience.

REACHING ECSTASY AND THE IMPORTANCE OF ORGASM

This might be the reason why you're practicing tantric sex period. If it is then great, and here, we'll discuss the tantric orgasm in its entirety. It's a little more in-depth than you'd think it is, and it's something that can change your life for the better.

WHAT IS IT?

When we talk about the orgasm, it's usually a taboo thing. Mentioning orgasms at the dinner table or with family is something that, unless you live in an open household, is something you either don't do, or you can't. There's a lot about orgasms that we don't discuss, simply because of the taboo nature of it. But, did you know that your sexual health, mental health, and your physical health can be affected by your orgasms?

There are many people who don't realize that not all types of orgasms are equal, and one of the most powerful ones is the tantric orgasm. That's because, it allows for you to achieve everything that you desire and help to undo all of the harm that manifests in your life, helping you get what you really want out of it.

The tantric orgasm takes your orgasm to the next level and is oftentimes called the full-body orgasm.

TYPES OF ORGASMS

You can have an orgasm that isn't just sexual. An orgasm is the sudden release of energy that's not sexual all the time in nature, but there are orgasms that do happen through sex.

A sexual orgasm is an orgasm that happens through the at of sex, and usually, it's the peak of your sexual energy. However, it can be on a different level too.

There is also the energy orgasm, which might be the sudden release of energy that's accumulated. Did you know that a seizure is a type of orgasm since it's the release of energies? Yawning is too, so you can actually suddenly release a bunch of energy, and many times, this is a sudden, uncontrolled release.

Have you ever felt a sudden burst of energy and then suddenly felt the low come back after a little bit? That's the effects of an orgasm in place since this is usually the sudden release of energy and then the sudden realization.

You can control your orgasms as well, and you can control this sudden energy as well.

Tantric sex is kind of the full-body orgasm that you can enjoy. It's the sudden blow-up, the explosion, and the release.

But the tantric orgasm is a full-on orgasm that frees up the body, and oftentimes it will re-sensitize the body when people are experiencing it. It's literally an orgasm that's so powerful you can't really hold it back.

THE VALLEY ORGASM

The valley orgasm is usually what we call the genital orgasm because it's mostly just around that arousal, where we feel the savoring flavor, the sudden rise, and then the fall and then back to normal. It's a very cantered form of orgasm, and oftentimes, once you expand it, the sensation can then go through the full-body, allowing you to feel that nourished and exhausted wave as you go along.

Full body, in contrast, is usually when you feel it throughout the whole body experience the power of the orgasm. Many times, people think this is just the whole body screaming, but it actually can make the sudden sensation of the orgasm flow away from the genitalia, penetrating your entire body.

It isn't always the screaming and writhing, it's the feeling of the sudden release of the energy, and it can affect how you feel afterward.

ORGASMING WITHOUT AN EJACULATION

The crazy thing about this is that it can cause men to orgasm without ejaculation. It's actually not very difficult, and the main reason why some men can do this is that the focus is off the genitalia, and it's more on the entire body, and you feel the full-on intensity, and from there, the sensation of the orgasm starts to spread through the body.

Why should you try to go for this type of orgasm? Well, we'll highlight the different kinds of physical, and mental benefits that come about as a result of a tantric orgasm.

THE BENEFITS OF TANTRIC ORGASMS

Tantric orgasms are different because they offer more than just a mere genitalia orgasm. Orgasms, however, do lead to a feeling of both euphoria and pleasure, which reduce your depression, stress, and anxiety levels, and help to naturally boost your immune system too.

Plus, orgasms that are tantric allow for you to burn a lot of calories, relax, and also release those tension points in the body, not just from the genitalia. If your sleep quality is suffering, you can always have an orgasm, and it will help with this. It also increases circulation within the brain and the body, leading to a sharper brain, and better mental clarity. It also alleviates pain, regenerates cells, and also reduces aging in the body too.

Orgasms also release oxytocin in the body, which allows you to have stronger feelings of intimacy. A tantric orgasm focuses on releasing a lot of this, improving the bond between you and your partner, and making the connection between both of out even stronger.

But, it's more than just a physical benefit, it also will help you in a spiritual sense as well. The big thing about an orgasm is, after it happens, your body opens up to a state where you're very receptive, and all of the parts of the body start to feel the flow of energies, and a tantric orgasm does this to the whole body, not just to the genitalia. It can align you in a spiritual and physical sense and allow you to increase the vibration of your physical and mental perspectives too, so it helps with blending each aspect of yourself into different ways. During orgasms, the awareness of your ego dissolves, so you attain a state of infinite nature, and that's why sex and orgasms are spiritual tools. Orgasms are one of the best ways to attain enlightenment and that's why tantric sex is so powerful. You become more vulnerable and excited, and you also feel a much higher sense of awareness, and this sexual practice can and will change you.

You can even manifest what you want in life through an orgasm. It isn't just the conception of children through sex, but it can be pretty much anything. What many don't know, is that the tantric orgasm allows you to manifest everything that you can possibly want in life through the practice of an orgasm. This allows you to fully focus on and experience the moment of your orgasm, and when you focus on this at such a deep, intimate level, you conceive everything that you want.

Remember that, when you do have an orgasm all of that energy that's been building up is then released, and you can practically shoot out all of that energy that you want and desire, causing a manifestation of whatever it is that you want into the reality of the moment, making it possible to pretty much-attaining everything that you can possibly achieve just through an orgasm.

Sounds a little crazy, right? Well you should understand that this is a process, and you want to manifest experience through this orgasm, and it can help release the negative thoughts, and you should definitely consider this form of orgasm to be one of the most powerful.

HOW MANY TIMES SHOULD YOU EXPERIENCE A TANTRIC ORGASM?

Well, that depends on how much you need it. Some people need to look at the energy that's there. Look at orgasms as a form of relieving the tension and reaching a higher state, and not just using them for an escape. Some people do use these solely to escape the harshness of our world, but that won't help you. That's not a healthy use of the orgasm, but if you do it in a way where it's healthy for you to do, and for you to possess, then you'll be much better off.

So, some people can have a tantric orgasm once a week. Some people, if they really need to align their spiritual energies might do it more often than anything else. The big thing to remember here, so that you have to do this for yourself, for what you want out of a tantric orgasm, and for your own personal benefit. Don't worry so much about how you do it, but instead focus on the process of doing it.

EDGING AND HOW IT BUILDS THE TANTRIC ORGASM

One way to bring about the tantric orgasm and the experience is to delay the orgasm. This is a way to push yourself into a higher rate of arousal, helping you experience the deeper, more forceful orgasms that can help you feel better, and reach towards the full body.

Delaying orgasms helps you feel the power of an orgasm, and it can be more than just a sexual orgasm in many cases, but a physical manifestation as well.

Edging is the best way to do it, and you can do this to yourself, or to your partner. For men, it is said to bring about very powerful orgasms, but it works pretty well for women too.

It is a way where you get yourself to the point of orgasm, and then stopping, and then doing this again and again. It feels amazing, it helps you achieve orgasm, and is a big part of tantric sex.

One way I like to do this is to try it on your partner, and from there, do it on yourself. Your ca does this, stop, and then switch it up, taking turns bringing one another to climax, sliding back down, and then doing this again, and finally reaching the finale after a bit. It's a good way to experience this type of orgasm, especially if you're someone who is used to always having quick orgasms. It's a good way to stimulate the body too and it can be a lot of fun.

This state that you get into isn't always just from your genitals though. The idea behind it is to feel the orgasmic state within your body. This is definitely a different feeling. An orgasm is a burst of energy flowing through the body, and you should understand that the orgasm doesn't always have ejaculation at the end of this.

The idea of it is to feel it in your entire body and let go of the idea that you have to always just feel it in your genitals. This pulls you into a deep, orgasmic state. It may not mean that you even have a writhing or any destabilizing with the sensation. The idea behind it is to feel the energies that come in, and the union of everything that's going on in your life. It's a way to be subtle with the way your energies are, and you'll know the orgasmic state. It's a burst of energy, but it doesn't always have to be a violent or very apparent thing.

It can be subtle and understanding that will help you awaken the orgasmic state within your body. It will allow you to experience exactly what you want out of tantra, allowing you to desensitize the body completely.

Sometimes the best way to figure out what you like from a tantric orgasm is to figure out what you like from your own body, and what type of energies you want to release from this, and some of the different faces of that. This can be a deep, lifelong journey that you may not realize you've got to embark on to truly understand, but understanding the different nuances of your body will change you, and you'll realize that there is a deeper, more effective form of orgasm that you will experience, that you will love. Tantric orgasms can change your life, and it's a way to look at the energy from orgasm in a completely different way, and in a way that'll allow you to fully understand

and get a good grasp on what you need to do to experience the lifelong effects of this amazing feeling.

DESIRES

esire is the first phase of the sexual response cycle of desire-excitement-orgasm-resolution. It includes both fantasizing about sexual activity and wanting to engage in sex. Desire occurs prior to feeling sexual pleasure and before tumescence, the increase of blood flow into the genitals.

Men, as well as women, may experience two sexual desire disorders. Hypoactive sexual desire disorder is a lack of interest in sexual activity. People who actively avoid sexual contact with a partner suffer from sexual aversion disorder.

Having sexual desire is an integral part of being a human being. It is a basic characteristic of every living person in this world, and it is something which even women are entitled to. After all, their bodies are capable of producing estrogens which are primarily responsible for the generation of sexual urges in women.

BUT WHAT IS SEXUAL DESIRE?

Sexual desire is basically the longing for sexual intimacy. It can be described in many ways. From holding hands to doing sexual intercourse, as long as it does give off sexual pleasure, it is considered desirable. In simple words, it can be referred to as libido.

According to several studies, the sexual desire or libido of women is relatively lower compared to the desire which men emit. This is because women are more concerned about the emotions that go with the act of doing sex rather than focusing on the act itself.

Hypoactive sexual desire disorder (previously called inhibited sexual desire disorder) should be diagnosed when the clinician judges the client to have too few or no sexual fantasies or no desire for sexual activity. Not only does such a person not seek occasions for sexual activity but also he or she does not take advantage of readily available opportunities. Since many people who meet this criterion are satisfied with the condition (one study suggests 20% of the population have the disorder), the diagnosis may be applied only if the low level of desire seriously troubles the individual or relationships.

Some people with low sexual desire may be interested in

one form of sexual activity or one partner but not another, whereas others are generally uninterested in sexual expression. Hypoactive sexual desire disorder usually begins in adulthood, after a stage of normal desire. Some clinicians claim that more men complain of low sexual desire than of any other sexual problem, and low desire often accompanies other sexual problems.

As the level of sexual desire is always judged in the context of a relationship, one person's desire may be low only in contrast to a partner's sex drive. For example, a woman's sexual desire level typically reaches a maximum when she is in her late thirties. If her husband is of the same age, his sex drive is likely to be declining. Consequently, she may complain of his relative lack of interest when his desire level is normal.

People with sexual aversion disorder actively avoid genital contact with a partner and typically find that the idea of such contact produces anxiety, fear, or disgust. Some people with this disorder avoid only genital contact but enjoy kissing and cuddling. Others shun all actions that are remotely sexual in nature. To avoid sexual situations, they may evade a partner completely, neglect hygiene, or become intensely involved in work or social activities, including a church. Sexual aversion is less common than hypoactive sexual desire and is more common in women than in men.

Some people with sexual aversion disorder may panic when they face a sexual situation, and the disorder frequently impairs a marriage relationship.

Both sexual desire disorders are explained by similar theories, but the studies on which the theories are based are often poorly designed and conflicting. Clinicians commonly point to emotional problems in the relationship, such as anger or fear, and argue that the desire problem is a symptom of a larger difficulty with the relationship. Others suggest that the low level of desire is causing the problems in the marriage, and perhaps both are correct.

Another explanation points to experiences in the past, suggesting such causes as parents who taught strongly negative attitudes toward sex, a repressive religious upbringing, sexual abuse, or rape.

Sexual desire may be inhibited by depression, obsessive-compulsive disorder, or various medications, including drugs used to treat high blood pressure or anxiety. When such factors are the sole cause of low levels of interest in sex, the clinician should not diagnose a sexual desire disorder.

Some people have low sexual desire because of fear of the consequences of sexual activity, including pregnancy, appearing foolish, or contracting sexually transmitted diseases (STDs). The aids epidemic has increased sexual avoidance among college women in particular.

Where the sources of the disorder can be identified, changing the behavior of the partner or even the situation may reduce the severity of the symptoms. Some sexual desire problems are due to poor hygiene or insistent sexual demands from the spouse, both of which may be changed with some effort and improved communication. If the fears of negative consequences of sexual activity are unrealistic, education about likely outcomes of sexual interaction may be helpful. In many cases, however, it appears that therapy must be directed at uncovering the underlying, hidden causes of the disorder.

Cognitive behavior therapy, which works fairly well for other sexual dysfunctions, has not been as effective with desire problems. A common cognitive strategy of people with desire disorders is to begin thinking about negative situations and worries whenever they face a sexual opportunity. As this strategy usually reduces anxiety about possible sexual activity, it is reinforced and thus very difficult to eliminate. Further, by avoiding sexual activity, people with these disorders have few opportunities to learn that they may enjoy sex.

WHEN WOMEN LACK SEXUAL DESIRES

But despite the leniency women show towards sexually related matters, the women's lack of desires is quite a big problem. Whenever women lack sexual desires, great stress and frustration takes over and it often leads to depression and too many insecurities.

WHY WOMEN LACK SEXUAL DESIRES

According to medical professionals, the interest of women on sexual activities is due to a variety of reasons. Generally, it could either be due to physical differences or psychological problems.

Most of the time, women lack sexual desires due to the limited production of estrogens. Estrogens are basically the hormones produced by the female human body which is primarily responsible for generating one's sexual urges. Usually, this situation may be due to the medications women take; particularly birth control pills.

There are also diseases which may trigger women to lack sexual desires. Some of it may be anemia, diabetes, and Hyperprolactinemia or overactive pituitary gland. More so, addictions may lead women to lose sexual interests. Drug abuse and alcoholism could definitely play a major role in the gradual decrease of interest women have on desires.

As for the psychological problems which make women lack sexual desires, the primary reasons would definitely be depression and stress. It is understandable that when a woman is under great pressure and anxiety, her attention would most likely be diverted to solving the problem rather than noticing her sexual needs. More so, it can also be considered that lose interests on sex due to failed relationships. This aspect is particular with the partner whom the woman is having sex with. When there is a problem between the couple, there is this great possibility that sexual desires and activities will be inhibited.

Psychological problems why women lack desires can also include their emotional backgrounds. Women who experienced sexual abuse during their childhood, or whatever experience which could trigger their fear towards sexual activities, are most likely to lose sexual interests compared to those who didn't experience those kinds of abuse.

Deterring surroundings may also be classified under psychological reasons why women lack sexual desires. Culture and traditions may be two of the major reasons why women have to suppress their desires.

Identity could also play a role in why women lack sexual desires. Latent homosexuality can affect it terribly, especially if the woman concerned has a partner from the opposite sex.

THE CURE FOR WOMEN

Basically, the cure for women who lack sexual desires depends on the reason why desires are inhibited. There are a variety of methods to do in order to get over this sexual disorder. If the cause is from the physical aspect, medicine intakes could be suggested. If it is due to some psychological problems, therapies would most likely be the remedy.

But whatever the cure is, women who lack sexual desires will only regain their interest in sexual activities if they help themselves regain it. As said, desires are part of human nature so women should not take it for granted. If there is a problem, it should be acted upon. Otherwise, life would never be the same again.

HOW TO INCREASE SEXUAL DESIRE

1. Everybody wants a happy marriage towards a loving, understanding and ideal family. And to achieve this ultimate dream, one must be open for some changes and must learn how to embrace The following points are helpful tips on how you can enhance sexual desire and rekindle marital relationships:

2. Maintain a healthy lifestyle. A healthy mind and body is a key to a more energetic and zestful playtime in bed. Specifically, enthusiastic sex among married couples is jump-started with more reliable and vigorous cardio and muscular endurance and flexibility.

3. Learn how to experiment, explore and play around. Sometimes monotonous and repetitive sexual acts and foreplays have become boring and unexciting; thus, making sex less desirable and motivating. Submitting oneself to your partner enables both parties to enjoy at your best and make the most out of making love. And with that, you also increase sexual desire if you tend to reinvent sexual positions, sexual acts and the like to satisfy and please your sexual partner.

4. Be sexually attractive and confidently beautiful - inside and out. When you have gotten what it

takes to be sexually attractive, you effortlessly seduce your partner-the most appetizing way to start an active "fight" on the bed. Be bold, daring and desirable in his eyes. When this happens, he can surely say no to you and your delightful looks. Truly, to increase the sexual desire of your partner must be your ultimate target. And by seducing him or her, you indeed succeed.

5. Get the proper motivation. Know your objectives and desires. Then, put everything into practice. You will never know how effective your techniques and how worthy your efforts are if you don't give it a shot. Increase sexual desire, stay focused and get moving. However, you should also bear in mind that too much sexual intercourse is not good either but zero or lack of sexual activities is even worst.

6. Stay young, in love and inspired. Being motivated and stimulated, you also need to be an inspiration to your partner. Most of all, you have to redefine sex as an act done out of love, intimacy, and romance. The main key here to increase sexual desire is to stay passionate, gentle and intimate lover on the bed. Private times with your lifetime partner can be the best intimate moments with him or her.

Needless to say, do a self-check today and begin to increase sexual desire. Through this, you can be able to maximize your time and resources making your improved sexual activities more exciting and fun. After all, the above-mentioned tips on how to increase sexual desire are already presented to you and all you have to do is to put them into practice. So, to all couples out there, make love and do it just right, in satisfying moderation. Have fun and savor each experience!

POSITIONS AND TECHNIQUES

R ight now, will find out about various Tantric sex positions and procedures that you can use for spicing up your sexual coexistence.

THE SIDEWINDER

This position is enlivened from the yoga position of a similar name, and this procedure takes into account deep entrance. It likewise accommodates the couple to keep in touch. For playing out this method, the lady should rests on her side and supports the heaviness of her chest area with the assistance of her hands. She should lift one of her legs and place it on her darling's shoulder while the other leg is lying on the bed. A variety of this equivalent position is that then again the man can rests behind the lady and enter his partner from behind.

THE YAB YUM

The Yab Yum position is viewed as probably the best situation for having tantric sex. It is a genuinely simple situation to perform, and it takes into consideration synchronous climaxes. This position helps in animating quite a few places. Likewise, the man's hands happen to be free right now, he can touch his darling's body however he sees fit, since the couple would confront one another, it takes into consideration enthusiastic kisses also. The man should sit leg over leg on the bed or some other agreeable surface and hold his back straight. The lady should straddle him and fold her legs over his lower back. It takes into account delayed here and there developments that can help the couple in accomplishing an all-around planned climax.

THE LATCH

This posture permits the man to get a decent see his sweetheart's face and the other way around. This is an extremely attractive posture and aides in pleasuring both the partners. For playing out this procedure, the lady should be situated on a high stage like a table or even the kitchen counter. She will then need to recline and adjust her upper middle and her head with the assistance of her hands by inclining onto her elbows. The man should remain between her separated legs and enter her. This is one represent that doesn't need to be limited to the room and is ideal for an off the cuff cavort.

THE BUTTERFLY

This method is accepted to allow both the partners to achieve a significant level of rapture and takes into consideration deep entrance. For playing out this system, the young lady should rests on the table so that her butt lies at the edge of the table and the man should help lift her lower back marginally off the table and afterward place both her legs over his shoulders. Her vagina would be free for him to infiltrate while remaining in the middle of her legs. Since her legs are shut together, this fixes the vaginal waterway and gives a tight fit. The man should enter her while her butt is in midair.

THE DOUBLE DECKER

This is an amazingly suggestive posture and will help in accomplishing a climax no problem at all. The man will likewise be given a decent perspective on all the activity that is going on down there, and his hands will likewise have unlimited access to lay with his sweetheart's butt. This position is very enabling for ladies since they have all the control here. For playing out this system, the man should sit on the bed while his legs are collapsed under his body. The lady will then need to confront away from him and place her feet one either side of her darling while her feet are set level superficially to give her some help. When she has brought down herself onto his erect penis, then she will just need to begin moving advances and in reverse or can even decide on a here and there movement. The man should basically kick back and have fun.

THE LAST PLACE ANYONE WOULD WANT TO BE

This is an extraordinary posture since it permits both the gatherings to have a similar measure of control and ooze a similar measure of pressure for having a great sexual encounter. People will have equivalent balance right now. For playing out this represent, the man should sit on the bed and support his chest area with his knees. He will then need to move the lower some portion of his legs in reverse and place them marginally separated. The lady will then need to expect a similar position yet she will do as such while confronting ceaselessly from him and her run would be squeezing into his scrotum and her back against his chest. Her legs would be joined and afterward set in the space that is accessible between his legs and the man should enter her from behind. For this situation to be compelling, both the partners should remain as near to one another as could reasonably be expected.

SKIFF

This position is a slight adjustment of the lady on top position. Right now, bodies should be situated so that both the partners will find a good pace great take a gander at one another's face while occupied with the demonstration. For playing out this, the man should sit down on a seat that can marginally twist in reverse. The lady will then need to put herself on his lap and afterward place her legs on either side of the seat. The young lady should fire an allover development without anyone else, or her partner can help her by setting his hand under her bum and helping her move in an upwards and downwards way.

THE MERMAID

This is a somewhat fluctuated adaptation of the butterfly, and it takes into consideration a more solace and better hold. Right now, man can play with his darling's feet. Remember that feet are viewed as one of the most touchy and erogenous pieces of a lady's body. For playing out this method, the lady should expect a similar situation as she did in the butterfly, however her butt ought to be propped with the assistance of a pad. Her legs should loosen up and ought to be at a 90-degree edge. The man should stand near the table and infiltrate her.

TSUNAMI

This posture is very agreeable, and it is a sensual treat. This will knock your socks off. This posture is a slight alteration of the exemplary minister style. Right now, lady should expect the job that a man as a rule does in the teacher style. For playing out this, the man should rests level on his back, and his arms should be put close by. The lady should lie over him, and the man should embed his penis into her vagina. The lady should totally loosen up her legs with the goal that they are resting on his. Her palms ought to be put on his lower arm for giving her some help. The lady will then need to begin moving her pelvis in an upward and descending development.

LAP DANCE

This is a great posture for a man to encounter his darling's body in the entirety of its magnificence. His hands will be allowed to meander around her body, and he can do what he needs. The lady will face away from him as she would have, had she been giving him a lap move. For playing out this represent, the man should sit down on a seat, and his back should be kept straight. The lady will then sit on his lap and parity herself by setting her hands on his upper thighs or even his stomach. She will then need to lift herself gradually and place the backs of her calves and brings down herself onto his penis. Another variety of this would be that the lady should bring down herself onto his penis while confronting her darling and this will give him a serious decent perspective on her bosoms. He can choose to prod and play with them for whatever length of time that he satisfies.

PRETZEL

This is another represent that is satisfying to take a gander at and even simple to expect. This will cause the couple to feel incredibly attractive. For playing out this procedure, the couple should stoop before one another. The man should move advances, and the lady will fold her arms over him. The lady will then lift herself up and place her left leg by her darling's correct foot; her foot will confront downwards. The man will then need to put his left leg close to her correct foot. When taken a gander at a couple occupied with this posture, they look like a pretzel, an extremely provocative and mouth-watering pretzel.

THE SPREAD

This is an essential and an amazingly hot position. This permits the lady to get incredible delight since it lets her stroke her sweetheart and permits him the entrance to joy her. For playing out this system, the lady should sit at the very edge of the couch or even the bed and spread her legs separated. The man will then need to remain in the middle of her legs and infiltrate her. She can draw nearer to him and kiss him while his hands have the entrance to her full body.

THE ENTWINE

This posture looks intense and about difficult to copy, however then it very well may be pleasurable if it's done appropriately. This posture is tastefully engaging. For playing out this strategy, the couple should sit near one another and face each other. The man should put his legs on either side of his partner. The lady will then need to lift both of her legs and place them on either side of her sweetheart's sides, under his arms. The man's upper arms will secure the lady's legs, and the lady will then need to lift her upper arms and place them over his elbows. The man will then lift his legs and place them over her hands. This does sound very muddled, isn't that right? All the exertion that goes into it will merit your time and energy.

THE G-FORCE

This is maybe one of the most blazing tantric sex presents there is. This is the piece de opposition of all sex presents. The man has full oversight over his darling right now, both the people included will get extraordinary delight from this posture. For playing out this position, the lady should rests on her back on the bed, and the man must bow by her legs. He will then gradually lift her middle off the bed so she's offsetting herself with her head and her shoulders put on the bed. The man can either extend her legs at a 90-degree edge or infiltrate her, or he can likewise pull them separated and place her feet just beneath his chest and enter her.

THE WATERFALL

Right now, lady should put her hand on her sweetheart's penis and afterward let her fingertips brush his scrotum gradually and tenderly. It is a smart thought to use some ointment for making it progressively pleasurable. Her hands should be set on either side of his gonads, and afterward she should gradually slide her hands up till they arrive at the touchy tip of his penis. When this is done, the lady should give the man some time to chill off, and he will then need to respond the administration he got. The man needs to cup his sweetheart's vagina and touch all her delicate spots. He should slide his hands over her clitoris and her vaginal external lips.

THE SNAKE

For this, the lady should gradually extend the pole of her sweetheart's penis with one of her hands and let the other hand follow little circles directly under the leader of the pole. This is like giving a slow and delicate hand work. Proceed with these movements a clockwise way and afterward once you arrive at the leader of the penis move to anticlockwise heading. Keep this up for whatever length of time that your sweetheart can suffer it.

TANTRIC TRIANGLE OF TOUCH

The lady should rests on her back and spread her legs somewhat and twist them at the knee. The man will then need to embed his list and center finger into her vagina and marginally twist them upwards till they make a come here development. This will give the ideal incitement to her G-Spot. This will make her groan in delight. While doing this, he should put the palm of his other hand on her lower midriff and apply a little delight. This consolidated incitement will rapidly push her off the edge.

THE TEETER-TOTTER

There is nothing remotely guiltless about this specific teeter-totter. This is exceptionally suggestive. The lady should rests on her back on the bed, and her pelvis should be somewhat tilted upwards. A pad can be propped under her pelvis for doing as such. The man will then need to lift her feet and tenderly overlap them with the goal that her knees are laying on her bosoms and the bottoms of her feet are touching his chest. This position permits unhindered access to a lady's vagina, and the upward tilt will guarantee that he hits her G-Spot each time he pushes into her.

TUB TANGLE

Get your man to lean back in a tub that is loaded up with water and the lady should straddle him while her back is confronting him. When his penis has entered her, he should sit up so you both are confronting one another. Then she should fold her legs over him, and he will do likewise with the goal that their elbows are under their partner's knees. Clutch each other as firmly as you can and start an influencing to and fro movement. This allows for some enthusiastic kissing.

LOVE TRIANGLE

The lady should rests on her back on the floor or the bed and afterward she should lift her left advantage into the air. Her correct legs ought to be loosened up to her correct side, with the end goal that both her legs are lying opposite to one another. She will then need to move her correct hand and catch her correct knee and form a triangle on the bed with the use of her correct leg and her correct hand. The man should hunch a little and enter her while holding her knee. This position would give the man better pelvic control and furthermore the chance of touching from multiple points of view as you would need to. A slight variety can be added to this posture by requesting that the man pivot his hips in a roundabout movement while pushing into the lady; this will push the couple to their verge.

PRESENTLY AND ZEN

This posture can be used for giving a snapshot of relief from the approaching climax. Tantric sex isn't tied in with discovering speedy discharge; it is tied in with enjoying the experience. What better approach to do as such, than to control yourself directly before arriving at the final turning point. When you feel that it is possible that you or your partner is near climaxing, enjoy a couple of moments and reprieve liberated from the position that you both are in. The man can just roll onto his side and remain inside his partner at the same time. This position just requests a snapshot of break. Slow pushing is passable, however if you feel that, you are going to climax, then pause for a minute, delay, maybe appreciate a tad of kissing and touching before proceeding with where you had given up. This position gives the genuinely necessary closeness during the sex to make the entire experience additionally adoring and healthy.

TORRID TUG-OF-WAR

The lady should sit leg over leg on the floor or some other agreeable surface and afterward gradually sink onto his erect penis and fold her legs over his back. This position will permit the couple to confront one another and this implies you can grasp each other's elbows for offering some help and incline toward the bearing endlessly from your partner. This resembles playing a round of shy back-and-forth. If you both happen to be adaptable, then one partner can tilt their heads back and lean in reverse, away from the other partner. This position will take into account the arrangement of your bodies, and it will cause you to associate with your partner. It frames a close association and aides in gathering speed. Both the partners find a good pace player's right now the entrance can be controlled on the other hand by the partners.

THE PYTHON

The man should rests right now, his legs ought to be kept near one another while his arms are resting by his sides. The lady should bring down herself onto his penis and mount him gradually. When the man has entered her, then she can extend herself above with the goal that she's laying completely on his body. Both of your bodies would be superbly adjusted, and you can get a handle on one another's hands for gathering some speed and furthermore for offering some help. The lady will then need to gradually lift her middle off his with the goal that it nearly appears to be a snake that is ready to strike. She can push against his feet for including some greater development. You will both be touching each other completely, and her bosoms would rub against his chest, your hands would be gotten a handle on firmly, and his thighs would rub against hers. It takes into consideration deep entrance, however it additionally takes into account clitoral incitement. Since the couple would confront one another, this takes into account some enthusiastic kissing too. All the erogenous zones in the body would be animated.

IMPROVE TANTRIC SEX WITH THESE TIPS

The principle motivation behind Tantra is to assist you with accomplishing splendid climaxes that you have been precluded in light of the fact that from securing your standard sexual practices. Notwithstanding, this doesn't imply that Tantra ought to be dealt with daintily. Consider Tantra an erotic exercise. Tantric sex is viewed as more charming than going through hours together at the rec center, yet the measure of physical effort that your body encounters can be contrasted with that you may understanding while at the same time playing out any overwhelming activities.

Additionally, there are various degrees of Tantric sex. Essentially bouncing into Tantra with no experience or primer practice may improve your sexual coexistence, yet it is so much better when you participate in some type of pre-sex warm up practice that will help in setting the mind-set and working up some expectation concerning what is yet to come. There are a few manners by which you can heat up, however perhaps the most ideal way that could be available is give your partner a back rub and have your partner give you one also. This will extricate up your muscles, which is significant in light of the fact that solid muscles can hinder a full body climax.

The back rub that you are providing for set up your darling

for tantric sex has some particular standards that are joined to it, alongside a system that is intended to uplift the sexual affectability and make the body progressively open to assist sexual incitement. Additionally, this back rub can be combined with a procedure that can be used on a lady to cause her to accomplish a climax. This will contribute extraordinarily to the nature of tantric sex in light of the fact that accepting one climax makes an individual patient for the following one, and this furnishes you with the fundamental open door to coax your partner and draw out the sex.

THE USE OF OIL

The main thing that you need before you can give your sweetheart a pre-sex knead is oil. Oil is an incredible instrument that can be used if you need your back rub to be increasingly compelling. It helps in extricating the skin up and giving grease to your hands. If your hands can slide and coast easily over your darling's body all the more adequately, then it will likewise help in making the back rub increasingly sexy and causes in paving the way to the real sex!

The best oil that you can use in a pre-sex rub is grape seed oil. This is because grape seed oil has minimal number of individuals that are oversensitive to it, and can be incredible for your skin. In this manner, by giving your sweetheart a grape seed oil rub you will be helping him, or her get milder skin too, and isn't this a fantastic special reward? You can generally include a couple of drops of your preferred scented or basic oil to make the experience far and away superior. Distinctive fundamental oils can be used relying on the specific explanation behind which it is being used. For example, lavender can be used for unwinding and alleviating muscles; rose can be used for giving an increasingly erotic feel to the back rub.

If grape seed oil isn't accessible, go for whatever other oil that has been made with the end goal of back rubs.

THE TECHNIQUE

The primary thing that you should do is clearly begin spreading the oil over your sweetheart's body. Ensure that the oil is conveyed uniformly everywhere throughout the body, and remember that too little oil won't give sufficient oil and result in teasing. In any case, using an excess of would simply wind up getting chaotic, and this can be irritating. Attempt to locate the fair compromise! While you are spreading the oil over your partner's body, you will find that the skin ingests the oil rapidly. Thus, you should keep habitually spreading more oil over their body, if the grease quits being adequate.

When the oil has been spread over your partner's body, the back rub can appropriately start. At first, it would be a smart thought to begin with essential pressure of the entirety of the significant muscles. The muscle you ought to go for while applying wide and vague pressure are the thigh muscles since this zone is normally under the most strain for the duration of the day.

When the muscles have been relaxed up in your partner's legs, you can move their back, the second-most tense region of the normal body. Simply apply pressure with your straightened palm, and make sure to speak with your partner as much as you can about what feels better and what is excruciating.

Attempt gently slapping territories that you feel are as of now free to invigorate blood course in these zones. Recollect not to slap so hard that it harms except if your partner needs you to obviously!

When you have finished this back rub and released up the significant muscle gatherings, the time has come to start centered pressure with the tips of your fingers and your clench hands. There are explicit territories that you ought to focus during centered pressure, and these zones are determined in the following segment.

TERRITORIES
TO TARGET

Bosoms: The bosoms are one specific territory of the human life systems that will in general draw in a great deal of consideration, and it so occurs, that they are additionally an astounding wellspring of sexual incitement for some individuals. They likewise will in general have exceptionally thought purposes of strain that, when discharged, wind up causing the individual to feel fantastically loose and quiet.

Along these lines, bosoms are clearly going to be one of the most significant zones of the body that you should target. Purposes of pressure here are most likely going to be on the lower half of the bosoms. It is significant that you search, attempting to discover the zone where the pressure exists.

This little wad of strain can be discovered right beneath the areola, and your partner may likely shout out when you hit this specific spot. In any case, don't confound this torment and stop the back rub. This torment is entirely charming, with numerous individuals contrasting it with the inclination once gets while scratching a tingle.

Something imperative to note while performing such a back rub is the source of these little wads of strain that are available in the body. They are not just strong pressure. Their root is more mystical than physical in nature.

You are as of now acquainted with the different chakras present in the body. In any case, you most likely don't know that these chakras are the significant stops in an immense system of energy that is streaming inside your body, vortices through which energy continually streams. However, there are sure circumstances where the progression of energy can get disturbed.

This typically occurs because of a less than stellar eating routine or a physical issue in a previous existence that may residually affect your body right now. Therefore, when you apply profound strain to these points the energy begins to get discharged, consequently expelling the impediment that was formerly hindering the progression of energy in your body.

Discharging energy is agonizing and yet very charming in light of the fact that the progression of energy gives essentialness and expanded sexual affectability to your body. This implies when you knead these points, your partner is going to feel an extraordinary tingling vibe that will regress into a stimulating sensation as the blockage is expelled from the energy pathways in the body.

The most ideal manner by which you can apply strain to this specific point is by pushing down using the tips of your fingers. Start by applying pressure and moving your hands in a round movement. This will discharge the energy blockage in a mellow and proficient manner. The round movement extricates up stuck energy and afterward permits your hand to move away to an alternate piece of the blockage, permitting the relaxed up energy to stream into the energy pathway without being impeded by the pressure of your fingers.

You can likewise apply serious strain to this point. This is exceptionally valuable since it will discharge energy from the blockage in a very serious way, and this will wind up opening your partner up for extraordinary sexual incitement.

Butt: This is another zone of the body that a great many people are stirred by. For reasons unknown, the butt is similarly as inclined to blockages in energy as bosoms seem to be, most likely in view of the extraordinary sum strain they experience when the individuals they are appended to spend by far most of their day sitting in an office. With the measure of sitting that we do, it is no big surprise that the pathways of energy in our derrieres wind up getting sponsored up.

The significant thing here is to feel your way around the territory. Blockages can happen in a few distinct pieces of the butt, so you should look around a little to discover where precisely the blockage has happened. An odd little fortuitous event is that the energy blockage is likely going to happen in a similar spot on the two cheeks, so if you discover the spot on one cheek basically begin squeezing a similar spot on the other cheek also.

Apply a similar round movement with the tips of your fingers that you used on your partner's bosom. These energy blockages may require some more pressure, notwithstanding, so if your partner can't feel anything when you are rubbing that person, simply having a go at using your thumb.

You may confront trouble finding the pressure point right now the body, particularly if your partner has been skilled with a breathtaking posterior. This is because the energy pathways are covered underneath a great deal of substance. Bosoms once in a while ever posture such an issue, regardless of whether the bosoms being referred to are very huge.

This is because the pressure points situated in bosoms are not as profound as the ones in the rear. Henceforth, if you are confronting troublesome finding your partner's pressure point, use your thumb, and it will work. If your thumb is as yet not adequate, have a go at using something inflexible like a pen to apply pressure, simply ensure you use the backside of the pen and not the pointy end!

Using such a device will assist you with providing unimaginably engaged pressure onto the energy blockage, encouraging a speedy scattering of energy and in the process most likely turning your partner on a lot.

Internal thighs: Finding the blockage in energy right now your body may end up being significantly more troublesome than discovering it on different pieces of the body. This is the reason a cursory back rub of the thighs is important before you start to test for pressure points.

The muscle rub is useful in light of the fact that it will expel a great deal of interruptions from that general region. A great deal of the time, you may be examining for the pressure point and would as far as anyone knows think that its rapidly, just to find that it was simply fundamental muscle torment and not the agony that originates from a blocked energy pathway.

However, if you have loosened up the muscles in your partner's thighs, the procedure ought to be significantly simpler. One great tip that you ought to follow is to search for the pressure point in the upper internal thigh, which implies the territory of your thigh that is legitimately beneath your partner's groin.

Attempt to crush this zone for the most part to locate a general area of the pressure point, and afterward slender it somewhere near using the tips of your fingers. When you discover the pressure point, begin applying a similar roundabout pressure that you used to both the past body parts.

Be careful while applying strain to the internal thighs. The pressure point here is significantly more sensitive than the pressure points in the butt or even the bosoms. Delicate pressure will take care of business, and apply an excess of pressure will simply wind up causing pointless agony that will likely power your partner out of the temperament.

If the round movement strategy ends up being unreasonably extraordinary for your partner, have a go at pushing your fingers ahead as you delicately knead the point. This will help by applying a lot gentler pressure than the roundabout movement, and the way that it is significantly more arousing absolutely doesn't hurt either!

Lower back: This territory of the body is totally different from the three zones talked about beforehand, thus will handle in a way that is totally unique to how that the past body parts were handled

What makes the lower back so one of a kind is that it doesn't have a solitary purpose of energy blockage that you should concentrate on. Or maybe, your partner will have one of two potential energy blockage circumstances, every one of which has its particular system that you can use to handle it.

The principal circumstance would be that there are a few dozen separate purposes of energy blockage that are peppering over your whole lower back, being centered explicitly around the segment of your lower back legitimately before your butt alongside the region of your lower back that is straightforwardly along your spine.

The subsequent circumstance would be that the energy blockage would be spread out over the aggregate of your lower back, with the energy nexuses interconnecting to shape a system of blockages like the genuine system of energy pathways that your body has.

The subsequent circumstance is regularly found in ladies with huge bosoms and individuals who do a great deal of physical work. This is because such individuals will in general put a great deal of strain on their lower back, compelling the energy pathways to get blocked in light of the fact that these strenuous exercises would intrude on their flow.

By and large, the lower back is continually going to be

an intense spot of energy blockage except if your partner gets customary back rubs, and the advantage of this is even the scarcest back rub right now significantly invigorate your partner and will bring about practically moment excitement whenever done right.

To discover which of the two-energy blockage circumstances your partner is experiencing you will need to test a considerable amount. Use your fingers to see where the energy blockages are. If there are spaces between the points where your partner feels torment, this implies the energy blockages that your partner is experiencing are isolated from one another.

Nonetheless, if every last bit of your partners spinal pains when you rub it in that extraordinary bothersome, tickly way, then your partner's energy blockage circumstance is of the subsequent kind.

The principal circumstance is significantly harder to handle than the subsequent circumstance. Since the energy blockages are not associated, you will need to handle every one independently as opposed to all simultaneously. This is because endeavoring to knead a few points without a moment's delay could bring about terrible agony for your partner.

In any case, settling this energy blockage circumstance isn't that troublesome once you get its hang. Just press each pressure point and discharge the blockage by moving your hands in the roundabout movement that you will be recognizable to at this point. You will before long find that once you deal with one blockage, the ones around it will start to get more fragile consequently.

This implies concentrating on a few significant spots will permit you to scatter the energy blockages and have the energy pathways streaming openly in the blink of an eye.

The subsequent circumstance, in any case, requires an altogether different methodology. The main thing you should think about this methodology is that it includes positively no nuance. The energy blockage is serious and will hinder your partner's climax, and since the blockage is across the board and interconnected, the best thing that you can do is attempt to handle at quite a bit of it simultaneously as you can.

Warm up your partner's lower back by using your thumbs to slide the energy blockages into getting somewhat more fragile. Following a moment or two of this, you should start using your clench hands. Ply your partner's lower back as though it was batter. This may appear to be clever, however if you ply your partner's lower back precisely how you would massage mixture, with the snappy developments and not remaining in a similar spot for a really long time, your partner will before long be loose to such an extent that they'd feel as if they are drifting endlessly.

The subsequent circumstance, albeit in fact increasingly serious, is significantly simpler to disperse than the primary circumstance. Simply ensure that you don't wind up harming your partner by applying an excessive amount of pressure. Keep in mind, correspondence is fundamental if you need to ensure that the back rub experience is as pleasant as could be allowed.

You will find that no other zone will give as a lot of sexual incitement as the lower back as it is being rubbed. This is because the energy that is being discharged is making them much progressively touchy to sexual improvements. Giving your partner a full body climax will turn into significantly simpler after you have rubbed her back to the furthest reaches conceivable.

CONSIDERATIONS AND FACTS ABOUT TANTRIC SEX YOU SHOULD KNOW ABOUT

Tantra has some wonderful components to it, and a lot of people should consider using this. But there are a few considerations that you should have in mind before beginning the tantra path.

YOU MIGHT NOT GET IT RIGHT THE FIRST TIME

This is a big one because a lot of people think you're just going to have hours and hours of mind-blowing sex, but the truth is, you might not even go ten minutes with the other person. It's a type of practice that requires patience, and you should always set aside the time you spend with your partner for tantra. But, always understand that it might not be done right the first time, and you might not even get it right the second or third time. This is like anything else, you need to realize that it takes a bit for you to really get the right feelings that come from this, and that, with tantric sex, and it takes a bit of time to really feel this type of connection.

REMEMBER TO GET
RID OF HAVING PLANS

This is something I always forewarn everyone with tantric sex. You need to have a plan in order to get into tantric sex. Having plans when you're doing tantra is both good, and not so good. You need to realize and understand, and you have to realize that, with the right mindset you'll get more out of this.

Our lives are very ingrained in making sure we get to X, Y, and Z, but we need to experience the fun of the moment, and you need to realize that while plans are good and all, get rid of the obsession with having them, and you'll realize that, with each passing moment it will make everything better. Having plans is nice, but it's also good to make sure to have a realistic, understanding mindset of what it is that you need to do, and everything that's in place. If you go into this obsessing over the goal, it won't work.

IT'S A POWERFUL TECHNIQUE

While you're probably doing this for sexual fulfillment, one of the biggest things to remember is that tantra does work with strong energy. The sexual energy that's exuded with this is usually sublimated which means it creates a higher level of consciousness, but it is very strong, and it can do a lot of things.

Tantra is powerful, and you should make sure that you do meditate before you consider this action.

It is oftentimes a practice that most people don't realize isn't something that you should be jumping into. That's why we encourage you to do yoga, detox and purify the mind before you continue. Sometimes, when people engage in tantra, their sexual energies increase too soon, and so do their negative qualities. Sometimes, with tantra you might feel angrier sometimes, and sometimes, you need to understand that, if your mind isn't clear and you're not just focused on the other partner, it can manifest things you might not be ready for.

While this is more with the ritualistic path of tantra, that doesn't mean it may not happen to you. Sometimes, people don't realize how powerful this technique is, and that, the energy that you're working with is very potent.

WORK TOGETHER

When it comes to tantra this isn't a one-person party unless you're doing tantric masturbation. The goal of tantra is to be able to work with your partner together to achieve the ultimate pleasure and make the other person feel good. But you don't want orgasm as the goal. You should work together in order to make yourself both happy and satisfied. This is something a lot of couples miss at times. They go in only thinking about their goals of trying to get the other person off or giving them the tantric orgasm when it's the process that means a lot more than anything else. So, don't be afraid to make this a mutual thing, and don't be afraid to make this work, and try to create a synergy behind it. That way, it will help with the pathway that you take, and you should always make sure that you're willing to do that.

MAKE SURE YOU'RE IN GOOD PHYSICAL HEALTH

While tantra doesn't focus as much on the health of a person, it's good to be in good physical, and mental health before you try this. That's because, it can take a bit of time before the results come about, and if you're not both on the same page with this, it can pose problems.

Don't think you have to be some star athlete though when doing this. The idea behind good physical health is that you at least have some sexual stamina and health, and you feel physically good. That way, you're happier and better than before. This is the way you should compose yourself when doing tantra, since physical and mental health are both very important, and you should always make sure that you can handle the effects of tantric sex before you begin.

If you've been at risk for illness and injury before, make sure to see your doctor before you begin with tantra, and if there are any medical conditions, get clearance before you start with this. It is a bit of an important thing since most don't realize the sheer impact of tantra on the body. It's very powerful, so make sure you're ready too.

NO DISTRACTIONS DURING TANTRA

Finally, try not being distracted during tantra. Of course, this is again easier said than done. But you should treat tantra as a sacred moment, which means that you're going to experience a lot of calmness of the mind, and a lot of racing throughs disappear.

His can be scary for those of us who are always worried about things, always stressed, and unsure about this.

Oftentimes, if we're overstimulated, it can affect the way your tantric experience goes. For a lot of people, the right tantric experience will change the way things go, and you have to, with tantra especially, understand that this energy isn't a toy, and it's not something to lay around with.

The distractions should be minimized. Keep electronics and other distractions out of the room during tantric sex, and you should go into it with a peaceful, calm mind. That's why we encourage you to do breathing meditation before you begin since if you're breathing evenly and calmly, it can help with keeping you grounded, especially when dealing with the energies, since they're strong, and it's better if you take the time to properly understand and fortify your own personal wellness with your energies, and the tensions that are there.

Tantra is a very fun thing to do, and it's a wonderful way to bolster the connection between you and your partner but you must understand the effects of it, and the cautions you must take with tantra. The right mindset will change your life, and you should, with tantra especially, understand the impact of it over time, and the effects of it as well.

CONCLUSION

Tantra is the ultimate love affair with yourself and all of your existence. In the process of igniting your internal flame, you come to experience all ordinary moments as extraordinary experiences. Immersed in the experience, you realize that you are the divine, there is nothing else to need or want, but that moment. The Tantra is thus a great movement for the uplift of human existence, for the recovery of the whole of man to god. All life is sought to be spiritualized and given high value as a field and means for the manifestation of the divine. Not only in its aim but in its method too. The Tantra seeks to extend the claim of the spirit on all the members of the society. The special characteristic features of Tantras are that they are extremely liberal and open to all castes and both sexes without any restrictions. This catholicity of the Tantric religion stood on the one hand against the Vedic practices and the metaphysical philosophy of the Upanishads and on the other, controlled the general mass by the force of energy of its magical appeal. In general, it is an attempt to point out that the tantric practices serve the function of helping practitioners to achieve a state of pure concentration.

Tantra art is based on rituals, which includes Yoga, offerings. Meditation and sexual intercourse. The most important concept found in the Tantras is the necessity of unifying apparent opposites in order to attain enlightenment. These opposites are usually represented as male energy (Shiva) and female energy (Shakti) or as the individual (Purusha) and nature {Prakriti). This the equality, or complementarily, of male and female, is a foremost aspect of tantric practice, as the union of both is required in order to achieve the highest understanding.

Tantra lies at the nexus of a series of conflicting extremes—the archaic past and the modern age of darkness; sexual liberation and sexual depravity; political freedom and political violence— each of which is seized upon in different historical moments. Perhaps most importantly, we have found that the image of Tantra has progressively shifted from a tradition associated with secrecy, danger, and occult power to one associated primarily with sexual liberation and physical pleasure.

Tantra is not something meant to be read about in books. What the text consists of are prescriptions for action including mental action which are the whole purpose of the texts. If you don't do what your Tantras describe, then you will never get the point.

It's an exact series of steps that allow and provide to others the wellness and understanding that you should have wit yourself, and with others. Tantric sex is one of the best ways to bolster the relationship that you have with the person that you love, and if you feel like you could benefit from tantric sex, then try it.

This is a beginner's guide to understanding the power of tantra, what it is, and some of the important factors associated with this, and some of the different factors that go into tantra. The right mindset for tantra will change the way your body handles all of the different aspects of tantra, and you should understand that, with tantra, you'll feel amazing, but you should also understand that it is a powerful technique, and it can change you.

With that being said, the next step for you to take is simple. That is to try out tantric sex with your partner. You can start out small by trying out breathing and going for about ten minutes or so and work up to it. Try using tantric sex in the bedroom with some of the small techniques that are there or the positions that are associated with this. With tantra, anyone can do it, and we provided the steps for you to get started on the pathway to pleasure though this type of sex.

www.ingramcontent.com/pod-product-compliance
Lightning Source LLC
Chambersburg PA
CBHW070705250726
48662CB00001B/265